Lots of Love!!

What Just Happened?
The Line

An *American Ninja Warrior*

Walk-On-Line Experience

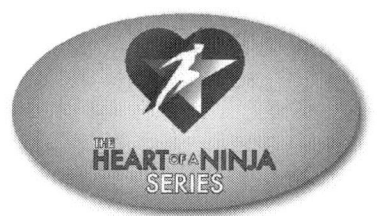

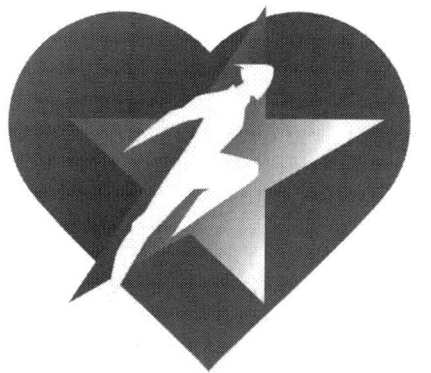

Also by Chris Warnky

The Heart of a Ninja: Stretch Your Boundaries

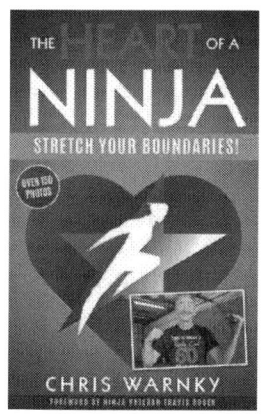

What Just Happened?
The Line

An *American Ninja Warrior*

Walk-On-Line Experience

Chris Warnky

Well Done Life LLC
Columbus, Ohio
2019

Well Done
Life

Copyright © 2019 by **Chris Warnky**

All rights reserved. No part of this publication may be reproduced, distributed or transmitted in any form or by any means, including photocopying, recording, or other electronic or mechanical methods, without the prior written permission of the publisher, except in the case of brief quotations embodied in critical reviews and certain other noncommercial uses permitted by copyright law. For permission requests, write to the publisher, addressed "Attention: Permissions Coordinator," at the address below.

Chris Warnky/Well Done Life LLC
1440 Mentor Drive
Westerville, Ohio 43081

Editor: Gwen Hoffnagle
Cover Layout by Fiverr pro_ebookcovers
Book Layout © 2017 BookDesignTemplates.com

Ordering Information:
Quantity sales: Special discounts are available on quantity purchases by corporations, associations, and others. For details contact "Special Sales" at the above address.

What Just Happened?: The Line
An *American Ninja Warrior* Walk-On-Line Experience/Chris Warnky – 1st ed.
ISBN: 978-0-9993331-3-6

Dedication

This book is dedicated to the thousand or more ninjas who have trained so hard and served time in an American Ninja Warrior walk-on line hoping to get a chance to run on the course.

It is also dedicated to the millions of fans who watch American Ninja Warrior on television or from the course sidelines – those who have wondered, "What in the world is it like to go through a walk-on-line experience to hopefully get a chance to run the course?"

"Wow, wow, wow, wow! What just happened?"

—Ninja Chris Warnky

Contents

Foreword 1

Preface 5

Introduction 9

Not This Year Either 15

The Numbers: *American Ninja Warrior* and the Walk-On Line 25

The Big Decision 35

Joining the Walk-On Line 45

Being in Downtown Cleveland 57

Finding a Place to Be 69

Cleveland Experiences 75

The Official *ANW* Line Forms 89

A Busy Sunday Morning 101

The Walk-Ons Video Shoot 113

Down to 30 Hours 119

I Have Learned So Much! 125

Photo Gallery 133

Learn More 155

Acknowledgments 159

About the Author 163

Foreword

Before I met Chris Warnky, I remember watching his daughter compete on *American Ninja Warrior* and, besides Michelle's strength and ability, I remember how emotionally charged Chris would get rooting her on during her run. As a father of a now 14-year-old son, I can only imagine the joy, nervousness, and overall pride that a parent must feel witnessing the greatness being displayed by one's own child. Chris definitely wears that for the whole world to see, and it is purely genuine. Now that I know Chris, I realize how excited he gets rooting on all of his friends as well. He loves the sport of ninja and the athletes who compete as much as anyone I know, and everyone in the ninja world knows Chris Warnky. He's made many friends throughout this journey, and I'm proud to be one of them.

I've also had the pleasure of watching him teach. As a teacher myself, I'm amazed at how naturally it comes to him. Chris teaches a Ninja Lite class at Michelle's gym (Movement Lab Ohio) for people who are beginning their journey and may be intimidated by the regular classes that have athletes with more experience and skill. With this in mind, Chris is a master at breaking skills down into simple steps and gradually progressing his students into more difficult maneuvers as they improve. Besides having the ability to instruct, he is also very supportive and positive. One of my favorite lines that he often says when somebody says they can't do a certain skill: "You can't do it, YET." In other words, keep at it, get stronger, and before long you will. Sometimes we all need a reminder that anything worth achieving requires relentless time and effort.

As I read *What Just Happened?: The Line*, Chris brought back many fond memories of our time together during the 10 days that I was in Cleveland and the thoughts leading up to making the decision to go. This is a great book for anyone to get that necessary nudge to make that leap of faith, to take that calculated risk, chase that dream, and prevent the feeling of regret later on. Even though things didn't work out the way I wanted, as Chris mentions eloquently in the book, I still value that chapter in my life and take out of it all the positive memories and relationships that were created. I haven't given up on my dream as I pursue an opportunity to get a chance to compete on the show.

I'm currently working on my application/video for season 11 in hopes of receiving "the call." Even though I know the odds are not in my favor based on the thousands of applications that are submitted, I have a realistic outlook and try not to let it get me down if I do not get selected. Even before I started ninja training, I was already going to the gym five or six days a week to stay in shape. Now I have more fun training in a group atmosphere with friends and doing obstacle course related training. Thanks to the NNL [National Ninja League] and UNAA [Ultimate Ninja Athlete Association], ninja competition organizations that have spread throughout the country have given many more ninjas a chance to compete despite not getting the call for the show. They even have an age group for the over-40 crowd so Chris and I don't have to compete against the young superstars.

One of the highlights of the book is the way Chris decided whether or not he should join the walk-on line. Too often we make important decisions based on what feels good at the time without considering the possible consequences. Chris put a great deal of thought into the pros and cons. He discussed it with his friends and especially his wife so he could be sure that he was considering all angles. I faced the same dilemma, and it just kept coming back to the regrets I would have if I chose not to go. I am very glad I went.

I now invite you to sit back and enjoy this crazy walk-on-line journey with us as you read *What Just Happened?: The Line.*

Ninja Scott Walberry

Preface

Have you ever had an experience that was so wild, crazy, and fun you just wanted to bottle it up so that you could keep it and not let it get away – you wanted to be able to go back to it and drink from it as often as you would like, over and over? That's how I feel about my Cleveland *American Ninja Warrior* walk-on-line and course-run experiences.

When I started on this path I wasn't sure where it was going to take me. It created a lot of surprises for me, some pleasant and some not so pleasant. I will never forget them.

Have you wondered what it would be like to go through the *American Ninja Warrior* walk-on-line process and eventually step up on that big, brightly lit stage? It occurs in the middle of the night, with the video cameras zooming in and out from every possible angle, while hundreds of on-site fans and potentially millions of TV viewers gaze at you, cheering for you to beat that course while the casting director and course producers are calling out directions for where and when you should make your next steps. That is a very memorable experience!

I have done it! In *What Just Happened?: The Line* I share the very personal and real experiences from the Cleveland *American Ninja Warrior* walk-on line. You are going to know what it feels like, at least from one 60-year-old's perspective. And I share the thoughts, emotions, and actions that led me to joining the walk-on line.

I had two primary motives for writing this book. One was capturing this unbelievable *American Ninja Warrior* walk-on-line experience so I can remember and relive it in my mind over and over again. It was fun and challenging, and I can still hardly believe I went through it. This book will help cement it in my mind for the rest of my life. I also hope you find this experience educational, enjoyable, entertaining, and even motivational. I hope it encourages you to take another step with a new experience so that you can see what new opportunities open for you.

I wrote the majority of *What Just Happened?* immediately following my Cleveland *American Ninja Warrior* course run. I wanted to capture my thoughts and emotions while they were fresh in my mind – while I was still riding so high from it.

To do this I had to stop writing my book about my ninja training experience, *The Heart of a Ninja*, which I was writing during my Cleveland walk-on-line experience. I thought that doing a quick brain dump to document all that occurred would take seven to 10 days. I soon found that it required a lot more time. I continued to write, and it took five weeks to document the majority of *What Just Happened?* I hadn't dreamed that it would take me that long to write about this 15-day experience, but it did – there was so much to capture. During those five weeks I wrote 57,000 words, which is equivalent to a 250-page book. This second ninja book was supposed to be shorter: not.

Once I was finally done with the brain dump I stopped and set this book back on the shelf so I could jump back into completing

The Heart of a Ninja. It took me most of the next five months to complete the reviews and editing, the book formatting, producing the cover, and finally publishing it.

The Heart of a Ninja is 240 pages of my heart, sharing how "I won" just by investing in my first three years of ninja training and competing. It also includes 12 traits of a ninja and a section sharing the stories of three female ninjas over 40 and 11 male ninjas over 50. I share many fun and interesting experiences that I hope will encourage and challenge you to live an even better life than you are living today. *The Heart of a Ninja* is available at Amazon.com.

In early 2018 I was excited about starting the editing process for the already written *What Just Happened?* It had taken several months to complete this step for *The Heart of a Ninja*, resulting in over 7,000 edits that made it better and more enjoyable for readers.

I was able to get a good jump on the *What Just Happened?* editing during the first two months, and then March 7th happened. At about 8:20 p.m. I had a serious "ninjury" while training. I won't go into the details, but the resulting concussion took me out of commission for over six months. During this time I could not concentrate on much of anything, but by mid-August I was able to get back to editing. I was so thankful to get back to working on completing and publishing this enjoyable ninja book.

What Just Happened? was originally going to be one book, but I decided to break it into two so they would be easier to read and less expensive, and so I could get the first one published earlier. After this one, about my *American Ninja Warrior* walk-on-line experience, my next and third ninja book, *What Just Happened?: The Run: An* American Ninja Warrior *Cleveland Course-Run Experience,* shares in detail what it's like to step onto the platform and run the course, and the highly emotional days that followed up through the airing of the NBC episode.

I believe *What Just Happened!* will give you a greater appreciation for the obstacles, skills, and abilities of the ninjas you watch run the course on TV. It is something else!

This was quite a ride that I have bottled for you in *What Just Happened?.* I'm confident you will enjoy it and feel a great deal of the emotion that I felt as I walked through each step.

Fasten your seatbelt. You are about to experience what it's like to be one of those "rookies" whom announcers Matt Iseman and Akbar Gbaja-Biamila refer to so often on the show. Through this book you are going to earn at least a part of your "ninja rookie" stripes as you join me in reliving my *American Ninja Warrior* walk-on-line experience.

Introduction

"What Just Happened?" Over and Over in My Mind

Wow! What just happened? Did I just join the *American Ninja Warrior* walk-on line and run the Cleveland city qualifier course? I think I did! Wow! I can still hardly believe it.

At times it still feels like it must have been a fantasy or a dream. It seems like it did not really happen. But when I look at photos from the experience I see my famed red "POM" sponsor towel, which all ninjas who have fallen in the water on the course are very familiar with, folded and sitting on my filing cabinet in my study; I see the little gift bag labeled "Dad" on the top of my bookshelf that came from Michelle at the front of the ninja course at the beginning of the night; then I say to myself, "I think this really did happen." When I slow down long enough to ponder this experience I just continue to repeat over and over in my mind, "What just happened?"

I never would have dreamed that it would happen in my 60th year on this planet, after 38 years of marriage, raising two kids, having two grandchildren, working in the corporate world for over 33 years, being retired for four years, being a part-time executive and life coach, and so much more. Could this really have happened, now, to me, an average guy? It did! And I'm so glad I joined the walk-on line. It really was quite the experience!

It's ironic that this book is being published with this title more than one-and-a-half years after my actual walk-on-line experience, but the title was just so fitting that I stuck with it.

A Rigid Guy Displays Flexibility

Throughout my life I have been a relatively controlled guy. I have many habits that I execute intentionally and routinely, every day. I'm a great planner. I think most things through very well and take most of my actions intentionally. One example of this is being able to retire at age 56, which was actually a little off plan. I had planned to retire at age 57, but circumstances allowed me to make that change even a little earlier. Some would say I live a pretty rigid life, successfully achieving the things I want to accomplish.

This is where *ANW* comes in, especially the walk-on line. This walk-on-line experience totally took me out of my routine and calculated world, and forced me to live moment by moment with whatever happened to surface at the time. There was very little planning during this 16-day period in the walk-on line. I think it was very good for me. I definitely saw things from a much different perspective.

I'm happy to say that I'm now back home and living my life the way I lived my first 60 years. It feels so good to be back to my normal, even though the walk-on-line experience was very good for me. It helped me see other aspects of life that many live with all the time. I now have a much better appreciation for at least one other type of existence on this planet. I'm thankful I had this opportunity. I'm a better person because of it.

It's ironic that I lived a good deal more of this unplanned life in 2018 as I dealt with my ninjury and the concussion that lingered for over six months. I was not able to be as calculated as I normally am. The goal for many days was just to survive and make it through another day while my body healed. In many ways this was similar to the mindset I had during my walk-on-line experience: survive and make it through another day. Maybe the walk-on-line experience was preparation for what was to come.

The Walk-On Line Is Not Easy

The walk-on process is not easy, which is why I had never considered it in the past. It takes a lot of dedication and you and your family have to be willing and able to make sacrifices in many facets of your lives. In the chapters ahead I share my experience of not only being a walk-on-line member, but doing it at 60, in the midst of a bunch of 20- and 30-year-olds. It was an experience.

The Journey or the Destination?

Years ago I had a boss who told me, "It was the journey, not the destination that was most important." For a number of reasons I did not get along very well with this boss. One of the reasons was my intense focus on goals and getting to a destination – to complete my goals. Now I have a much better appreciation for the concept of focusing on the journey more than the destination. We need both. Without a destination – a goal or dream – we don't strive or plan. I find that my days feel less meaningful if I'm not striving for something. I'm learning to "smell the roses" more often, to enjoy the process, and to embrace the journey along the way. I now find that the bigger my goals the less probability I have of achieving them. If I miss a goal it can be frustrating and depressing. By focusing on the journey I work much harder to appreciate the moments that pass and the learning and growth that take place along the way.

The walk-on-line experience helped me improve my focus on the journey. When I committed to go for it I knew there was no guarantee I would get to run on the course, and that I had better enjoy it and learn from the effort if I wanted to get something from it. This perspective enabled me to take the steps to join the walk-on line; create many new, fun, and challenging experiences; and eventually run on the *ANW* course. I am so glad I have learned to apply this perspective. I hope you enjoy this ride with me as I look back on my experience. I hope you are already better able to enjoy your ride in this life than I was. We have been blessed with so much, especially those of us who live in the United States of America. We have so much freedom. Don't take it for granted.

Do What Is in Your Control

I hope you come away from *What Just Happened?* encouraged to focus on what you can control rather than trying to control everything. We experience much in our lives that is not in our control, yet there is still a great deal that we can. These things steer our lives. Focusing on what we can control provides us with enough to keep most everyone I know quite busy. I believe your reading about my ninja experience will help make this point, and I hope it will be a model for you to take greater control of your life in the areas in which you have control. It can and will change your life.

Be Content with the Outcome

I also hope you see how important it is to be content with the way things turn out. We must focus on what we can control and learn to be content with the results from these efforts. Believing we control things that we don't is a formula for significant disappointment and disaster. I hope after reading *What Just Happened?* you choose to become even more content with the situations in your life that you don't control.

Take Another Step

Recently I was listening to a song by Steven Curtis Chapman. The song is titled, and repeatedly states, "Take Another Step." The key message is to keep going and not give up, give in, and stop. I love the message of the song. It reminded me of the core message of this book, which is "open a door, or another door, and discover more and new opportunities."

It is so easy to get stuck and not move or try something new. When we remain stagnant or stuck we lose the ability to see so many new opportunities. I hope that *What Just Happened?* is a great model of the new opportunities that can surface by taking that next step and opening a door. For you that might be a door that you have been standing in front of and staring at for who knows how long. I hope you step through that door to see what's on the other side. I'm so glad I opened a new door by getting in the *ANW* walk-on line!

The Structure of *What Just Happened?*

The chapters are mostly in chronological order, but I supplemented them with chapter 2 on *American Ninja Warrior* numbers and chapter 13 called "Lessons Learned." At the back of the book I provide a Photo Gallery. As we travel through this experience together, I hope these photos are fun for you and help you better appreciate what it felt like to walk through this experience.

Chapter 1

Not This Year Either

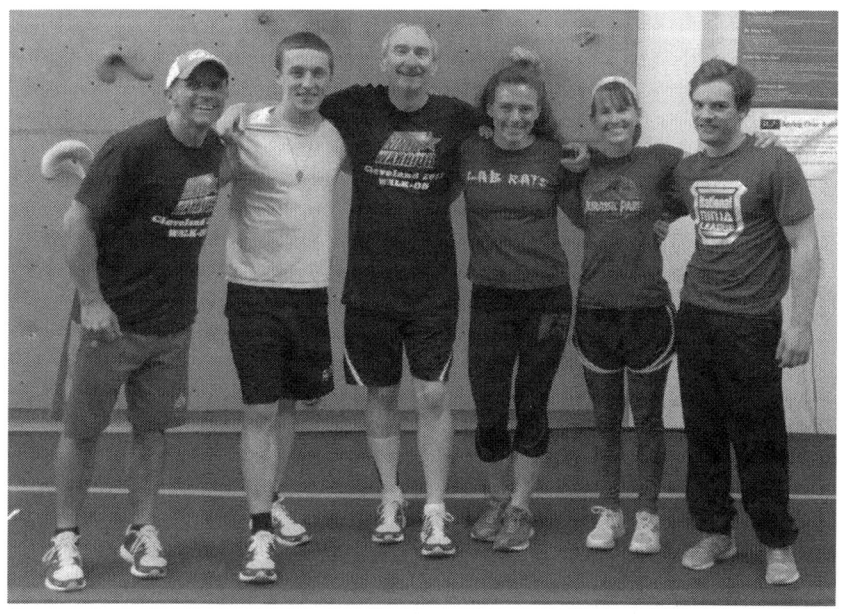

How did this all start? To compete on *ANW* you must complete an application and produce and submit a video. I did that in 2016 and again in 2017.

By April 20th of 2017 it was evident I was not going to get the call to compete in Cleveland that year. I had trained hard to represent myself well for the casting and production team at NBC but they must have had even better stories, personalities, and athletes to invite. NBC knows who I am. It was just not to be again that year. Two in a row. It was hard, and it was reality. I had gotten so much stronger and focused my submission video on me: my story, my personality, and my ninja skills. I intentionally worked not to make a big deal about being Michelle's dad, but still no invite.

I promised myself at the end of *American Ninja Warrior Season 8* (*ANW8*) in 2016 that *ANW9* would be my year to "play and have fun" on ninja obstacles. At the end of the year I would evaluate whether my skills had improved enough to produce a submission video.

To Submit or Not to Submit; That Is the Question!

During this time I captured a lot of fun videos of me playing on obstacles. As I reviewed the footage I saw how much I had grown in both strength and skill. With the encouragement of many ninja friends I decided to complete the application and produce another submission video for *ANW9*.

Unlike the prior year, when had I spent over eight months strategically capturing video of my training and competition experiences; written, rewritten, and edited my script; and recorded the narrative over a period of weeks, this year I spent one week pulling all the video together, writing the script, recording it, and editing it. In the end the video was not perfect, but I felt good about it. It was about me and my skill.

Based on feedback, I focused much more on who I am and what my inspiration is than in 2016. *ANW* is all about inspiration. I shared that my two primary motivations were to love and honor my Creator, and the tremendous inspiration I receive from my ninja community (my tribe). You can see my 2017 *American Ninja Warrior* submission video at https://www.youtube.com/edit?o=U&video_id=WPpOy_ju_Xo.

Extra Video Review

I reached out to the *ANW* senior casting producer and shared my video with him before I submitted my application. He gave me a good deal of encouragement, saying, "It looked great! Don't hesitate to submit it...really good." This was an extra step I did not take in 2016.

As in 2016 I submitted my application and video well in advance of the cut-off date. Many of the ninjas would be scrambling last-minute to get their videos edited and their applications completed. I hit the send button weeks before that critical January 2nd due date at midnight Pacific Standard Time.

I had done all I could do. Now it was up to the casting team, the producers, and the executive producers to review the tens of thousands of applications and videos and decide who the 90 to 100 Cleveland competitors were going to be.

Waiting and Waiting and Waiting

As in prior years, Facebook groups surfaced to share information about who had been invited to compete. I was a member of two of these groups. As the first calls started coming in and ninjas began posting "I got the call!" my heart again started pumping harder and faster.

During this period ninjas who have applied become hypersensitive to their phones ringing. You don't let your phone ever get out of your reach or far enough away that you can't hear it. Every telemarketing call makes you jump. "Could this be *ANW* calling?" Buzz, buzz, buzz. "Is this it? Drat. No. It's my mom calling." I love my mom, but during this short window of time when *ANW* is calling applicants, anyone but an *ANW* casting official seems like a letdown. :)

During the first few days the Facebook posts came rapidly and were so exciting, leading me and so many other ninjas to think, "Am I next? How soon will they be calling me?"

I got really excited because so many of my close ninja friends from Movement Lab Ohio (MLAB OH) got the call. I celebrated with each of them. There were my daughter Michelle, Josh Wallis, Shanon Paglieri, Katie Tennant, Peggy Hale, and eventually Sean Noel.

Others from Ohio who had been to our gym and had previously competed on *ANW* were invited, too, including Amy Pajcic, James Donald Wilson, Eric Woodruff, and Logan Broadbent.

There were also some newbies like ninja Naeem Mulkey who had just started showing up at MLAB OH. Wow, Naeem was impressive for a guy who had never been on ninja obstacles. He is a great athlete with a wrestling background, just like ninja Sean Noel. It was so fun to get to introduce Naeem to some of the key ninja obstacles including the slanted steps, the warped wall, the salmon ladder, and several of our balance obstacles. It did not take Naeem long to master his technique on most of these obstacles. He was all ears as he asked us to share with him anything we saw him doing that he could learn to do better. Talk about an excellent student; he got A's from us, and we shared many ninja obstacle tips and techniques with him.

Hearing about the invitations for so many current and new friends was exciting! I was happy and pumped, yet in the back of my mind I continued to wonder, "What about me?" No call had come.

The Calls Stop

After several days of excitement the calls started to drop off. No longer were people sharing, "I got the call!" That's when the questions started to form in my mind: "Are they done?" "Are they still calling?" "Are there still a few others who are going to get the call?" "Why aren't they calling me?" "I have a good story! They love my on-camera energy as a sideline fan. They know who I am. In my video I focused on what they wanted: my motivations. I have significantly developed my skills during the year. Why have they not called me?" The questions continued to echo in my mind and I could not get rid of them.

I was not the only one from our gym not to get the call. There were several others including Jesse Wildman, Rex Alba, and Scott Walberry. (I share more about them later in my story.)

Over the next few days a few additional people posted "I got the call!" and my hope, although flickering, would slightly rekindle for a few hours.

I was excited for all those from MLAB OH who were invited to compete, but I thought perhaps I didn't get the call because there were already so many representing our gym. I was so happy for each of them and I didn't want any of them to be left out. Maybe six ninjas from our gym were enough. That was a fantastic representation from MLAB OH!

I reached out to the senior casting producer again to see if he could share any information with me. Were they done? Was there still any chance I would get a call? There was no reply to my calls. I called six times and left messages twice, but no reply. I'm sure he was overwhelmed with calls from people like me.

The senior casting producer is a great guy and has a ton on his plate during this peak activity time. I know that during some of my calls he was in Kansas City executing their *ANW9* city qualifier. I had to be reminded of this by my daughter, as I had tunnel vision: "What about me?" There were probably hundreds of others like me calling to find out if there was still a chance to be invited out of the thousands who submitted applications just for the Cleveland competition. It must be an overwhelming job, especially during these peak periods. I can't imagine how busy it must be during those couple of weeks when a hundred ninjas are being invited to compete in one city while at the same time a competition is being conducted in another city. There was no way to respond to all of us.

Some of the invitation calls are highly coordinated because *ANW* wants to get video from a spouse or a friend when the invitee gets the call. I saw some of those live reactions when the calls came in. It was fun to watch the reaction of Shanon Paglieri on video when she received her call while being driven to a sign language class. Maybe the best was the reaction from Peggy Hale when she got the call. Her husband had pushed for a "game night" at home and set it up for after a draining work day for Peggy. Boy was she confused by the push for a game night, and when the call came she was totally surprised.

A Letter to My Family and Friends, Again

Eventually, in late April, I drafted and sent my "No call again this year" letter. It went to my Facebook family and friends.

As bittersweet as it was, I was again generally okay with not being invited. I had not intentionally and strategically trained. For the past 12 months I had played and had fun and had not planned to complete an application and produce and submit a video. It had been a last-minute decision. Below is the letter I sent to my Facebook tribe on April 21st.

> I do not expect to get to compete in the Cleveland *American Ninja Warrior* city qualifier this year. NBC invitation calls started several weeks ago. Many ninjas have been invited and I have not received an invitation

call at this point. It has now been days since I have heard about someone else getting a call. With having 50-70,000 applications submitted and only around 600 ninjas being invited, *ANW* does not inform you if you are not going to be invited. There are a lot of us out here (well over 50,000) who wonder and wonder for quite some time. I have come to the conclusion that I will not be getting the call this year. We are down to almost 2 weeks until the competition will be held in Cleveland.

This past year I did not train to compete in *American Ninja Warrior* in 2017. I gave it my all to be ready to compete in 2016, working for 2 years on my skills. This year my focus was on playing and having fun on ninja obstacles. I did that very well and had a great year. In that process, I did really grow my skills and strength, so I did go ahead and complete an *ANW* application/video for 2017.

I am very thankful for this past 12 months. It has been another great year of investment in my development as a person and athlete. I have had the ability to: learn and grow, meet so many great new people, deepen the relationships that I already have, create many new experiences together, and contribute to many others in a variety of ways. It has been a great year!

I am fine. I am very excited for so many of my friends who did get invited this year to compete on *American Ninja Warrior*. We have had a good number of ninjas invited to compete from Michelle's gym, Movement Lab Ohio. It is going to be a blast to get to cheer them on from the sidelines. I am also quite sad for many other friends who trained so hard and did not get the call this year. My encouragement to each of them is to stay with it and keep learning and growing. It is all for their own benefit.

Under my goal of playing and having fun, I am considering signing up as a tester for the Cleveland *ANW* course. That could be a great and fun experience. I do have some friends who are wanting me to join the walk-on line in Cleveland.

This year I have also started writing a book about my fantastic ninja training and playing experience over the past 3 years. It has really been a great experience. It also includes the experiences of 14 other friends who are ninjas ages 40 through 70. This has been a great learning, growing, and stretching project for me. I am hoping to publish it in either late summer or early fall of 2017.

Thank you for your friendship and support during my life journey: ninja and otherwise. You have been so encouraging and supportive. I have been so blessed! Thanks for being a part of my life.

Comments from My Facebook Post

Here are a few of the comments I received from my "not invited" post:

Beth Higginbotham Crosby 🖤♡🖤♡🖤♡😀🤗Such an inspiration!!

Mike Steele I don't know how in the world they haven't picked you the last couple years. Michelle's your daughter, you have an amazing and outgoing personality, and you've actually gotten pretty darn good at Ninja. Please don't give up on it. Would love to see you give it a go next year for *ANW Season 10* 💪🤜👊👍👍😄😁😄😁😄😁

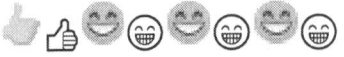

Brian Keane Wonderful words of encouragement and you definitely should try the walk on line since it is in Ohio. You're looking great and hoping to see you in Cleveland if I get the chance. Was great sitting and cheering with you in Vegas last year. Best of luck to your family and I will be pulling for **Michelle Marie**.

John E Loobey really cool shirt and a really, really cool guy!

Where Do I Go from Here?

My letter was sent. Where did I want to go from there? Should I show up and just cheer in Cleveland as usual or see if I could help test along with some gym friends who also did not get the call? There was the outside possibility of being a walk-on in Cleveland. If I did that I could be there for weeks. I had not given this option serious consideration, but technically it was an option.

Before I share my walk-on-line experience, the next chapter is about the number of ninjas who have competed and would like to compete on *ANW*.

Chapter 2

The Numbers:
American Ninja Warrior and the Walk-On Line

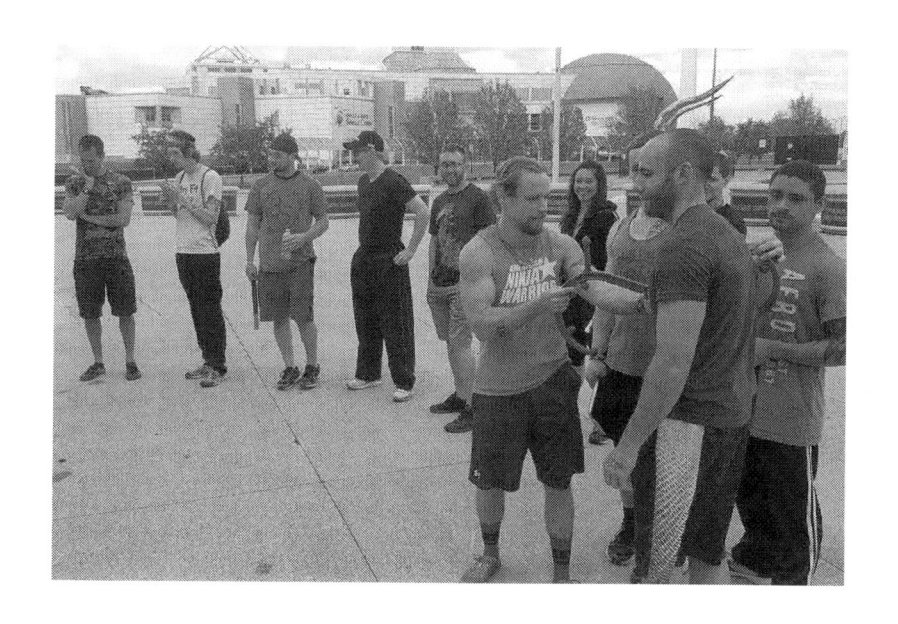

To provide some context, here are my high-level guestimates relative to the number of competitors on *ANW* up through season 10, or 2018, which was recently completed as I write this.

2,700 Ninjas

I'm not aware of the number of *ANW* competitors during the first three seasons, but let's say there were 100 to 200. Some of these ninjas competed multiple times during the first few years.

Over the past seven seasons there have been five or six city qualifiers. Usually about 100 ninjas get invited to compete in each city. That would be around 500 to 600 ninjas competing each year for the past seven years. That rolls up to between 3,500 and 4,200; so my initial guess was that there have been about 3,800 invitations to compete on *ANW*.

But each year a number of ninjas are invited back, so I'm going to guess that about 60 first-time ninjas are invited per city each year. That equates to about 350 new ninjas competing each year. Over a seven-year period the total would be about 2,500. If you add my guestimate of 200 ninjas from the first three years, there have now been about 2,700 ninjas who have been invited to compete.

Based on these guesses, I am relatively confident that somewhere between 2,500 and 3,000 ninjas have been invited to compete on the show through season 10, 2018. That means that there have only been 3,000 ninjas out of the 325 million people living in the United States — at most one in 110,000 people. Ninjas who have competed on the show are a very rare breed!

American Ninja Warrior Invitees per Application

Now let's look at how many ninjas are actually invited compared to ninja hopefuls who have "started" (in *ANW's* words) or completed an application. I read that in 2017 up to 70,000 people started an application. Since that's not an official number, let's assume that somewhere between 50,000 and 70,000 completed applications. As above, I assume that 500 to 600 ninjas are invited to compete in city qualifiers. That means that potentially 1 percent or less are invited to run on the course. That leaves somewhere between 49,400 and 69,400 ninja hopefuls each year who don't get invited to compete. This is truly an exclusive opportunity for those who are invited.

What Are the Other Options?

Thousands of ninjas each year spent countless hours training to develop their skills so they could compete on the show. What are the options if someone is not invited to compete? I am aware of four: join the walk-on line for a city qualifier; volunteer to be a course tester and hopefully get a chance to try some of the obstacles during testing (no TV exposure for this option); keep training for a possible run next year (and during this time participate in one or more of the ninja leagues across the U.S., like the National Ninja League (NNL) or the Ultimate Ninja Athlete Association (UNAA); and give up and just be a fan.

What Is a Walk-On Line?

Some ninjas try to get a chance to run the course by joining the *ANW* walk-on line. My depiction of the walk-on line is based on my experience in Cleveland in 2017. It's not an official description, just my perspective. I include information from other "walk-ons" in Cleveland and those who got in line at many other sites. Keep in mind that the experience can be different from city to city and from year to year.

The walk-on line is a self-regulated group of ninjas who show up at a course early enough to be considered potential course runners. Sometimes ninjas are required to stay at the site 24/7. In some places the city ordinances don't allow people to stay in line all night. And in others they are required to check in at designated times throughout the day.

First an unofficial line is formed that is regulated by the ninjas who have been at the site for days, weeks, or even a month or more before the competition. They create a list of their names in the order in which they showed up. To remain in their designated order they have to follow the rules they agreed to live by. The group selects a leader — the first or one of the first to show up, usually weeks in advance — and they monitor each other to ensure that each ninja is following each of the agreed-upon rules.

My Cleveland walk-on-line leader was in contact with the *ANW* senior casting producer to ensure that he was aware that a line had formed and who was in it. A few days before the competition an official walk-on line is confirmed by the senior casting producer.

Who Are the Walk-Ons?

Walk-ons are not the lower-class, weaker ninjas. They are often very strong ninjas who were just not invited to compete that year. They are usually very skilled and extremely dedicated. They are dedicated enough to go through the grueling walk-on-line experience to get a shot at getting to run the course.

Many walk-ons previously competed on the show. They might have had an early fall in a prior season, so were not invited back. They might not have submitted an updated story when they applied that, in the minds of the producers, would be of interest to viewers. There are many reasons a ninja would not be invited back to compete on the show.

Some of the top ninjas have been in a walk-on line, including Isaac Caldiero, James McGrath, David Campbell, Kevin Bull, Abel Gonzalez, Adam Rayl, Michael Silenzi, and David Cavanagh. And sometimes the walk-on-line ninjas who get to complete have never been on the show before.

The strongest competitors are sometimes not invited because the NBC personnel are not looking only for top skills and performance; they also want personality and great stories. If a ninja doesn't have all of these it's much harder to get invited to compete. *ANW* is not a competition recorded for TV but rather a TV show that includes a competition.

The walk-on line is one way to bypass the application process and get a chance to compete and build an *ANW* name for yourself. Some walk-ons have not even completed an application or provided a submission video at the time they get in line; they just decide they're going to give it a try.

Some Get in Line Year after Year

Some ninjas have joined the walk-on line year after year, and some have competed multiple times. For some reason they just don't seem to have all that NBC is looking for, so they don't get invited. To name just a few, these include my friends Julien McConnell, who was our walk-on-line leader in Cleveland, has been in line six years, and has had the opportunity to run the course three times; Greg Schwartz, who has been in line seven times over six years and competed three times; and David Cavanagh, who has been in five lines and competed five times, made it to four city finals and two Las Vegas finals, and made it to stage two once. David is one of the seven walk-ons who made it to stage two in Vegas. He was the last walk-on to get to run in his city in 2018. Yancey Quezada has been in line five years, in six lines, and had the opportunity to run four times. As you can see, sometimes a ninja will get in two walk-on lines in the same year if they don't get the chance to run during their first walk-on line for that year. They are all strong ninjas who have worked and trained hard.

What Are the Chances of a Walk-On Getting to Run?

Being in the walk-on line does not guarantee you will be given the chance to compete. In fact it can mean just about the opposite, because most walk-on-line ninjas don't get to compete.

There can be anywhere from 20 to 40 walk-ons in line. And I have heard that some walk-on lines included more than 100 ninjas all hoping to get a chance to run. That's a lot of competitors hoping to get a shot at the course.

My guestimate is that each year across the five or six *ANW* sites there are typically 200 to 300 walk-ons. Only 60 to 100 of them – just one-third or less – get to run the course. Everyone who joins a line knows the risk: they're not likely to run unless they're one of the first 10 to 15 people in line.

My understanding is that the number of walk-ons who get to run a course averages between 12 and 15. As of this writing the most that have been able to run in one night is 27; and the fewest is five, which has happened multiple times.

It seems that the way *ANW* uses walk-ons is primarily to kick off the official runs for that night, both at the beginning of the night and after the crew lunch break when they start filming again. If there is time at the end of the night, before daylight starts to appear on the horizon, they might run a few walk-ons.

If everything goes smoothly this can result in five to 10 walk-ons running at the beginning of the night, another five or so after the lunch break, and maybe a few more at the end of the night. Walk-ons compete only in the city qualifier runs. The city finals include only those ninjas who qualified.

If things don't go well and quickly on the night of filming there are fewer opportunities for walk-ons. Situations that can slow down a night include an obstacle breaking and having to be repaired; one or more ninjas getting injured during their course run; weather challenges like rain, heavy dew in the early hours of the morning requiring obstacles to be wiped down; lightning; high winds; and even a lot of ninjas who complete the full course, because that requires more time to reset more obstacles. When these situations occur, the odds of running many walk-ons drop significantly. It can be that only five walk-ons get a chance to run at the beginning of the night, which is heartbreaking for those in line. They are dedicated – waiting and hoping throughout the night – only to walk away disappointed to be so close but not get to run. The *ANW* crew works hard to provide opportunities to as many walk-ons as possible, but they're at the mercy of these factors as they work with the available time for that evening.

The lower a ninja's number in line, the better their chance of getting to run. Walk-ons one through five can be confident they will get a chance. Having a number from six to 10 is encouraging. From 11 to 19 you have big hopes but you know your chances are slim. Those over number 20 just hope that either it is an amazing night and many, many walk-ons are run, or that the producers will single them out to run regardless of their place in line; this can and has happened.

The producers have the authority to skip anyone and run someone further down the line if they feel it will make for a better TV show. There have been times when they ran someone with a higher line number because they learned something interesting about the ninja's story, they were wearing a particular costume, or any number of other reasons. The producers are in charge and it's their TV show; they do what's best for the show and their six million viewers. The paperwork ninjas fill out to compete, including those in the walk-on line, states that the producers have these rights, so it's not a surprise. That doesn't mean it's not a major pleasant surprise for someone and a big disappointment for someone else.

To summarize, there could be 30 ninjas in a typical walk-on line and potentially only 12 to 15 who get to run the course, or 35 to 50 percent. For walk-on lines with over 100 in line, and ones from which only five get to run, the percentage is 10 to 20 percent. The percentages are low, but many ninjas are willing to take that shot at running.

Not all of those in the walk-on line will have spent weeks in line. Many join the line just a few days before the competition when the die-hards have already been there a very long time.

I hope this overview allows you to better enjoy and appreciate my Cleveland walk-on-line experience. You have a jump start on me. At the time I joined the line I did not have this context; I was going to find out along the journey. Let's start this wild and crazy Cleveland walk-on-line journey.

Chapter 3

The Big Decision

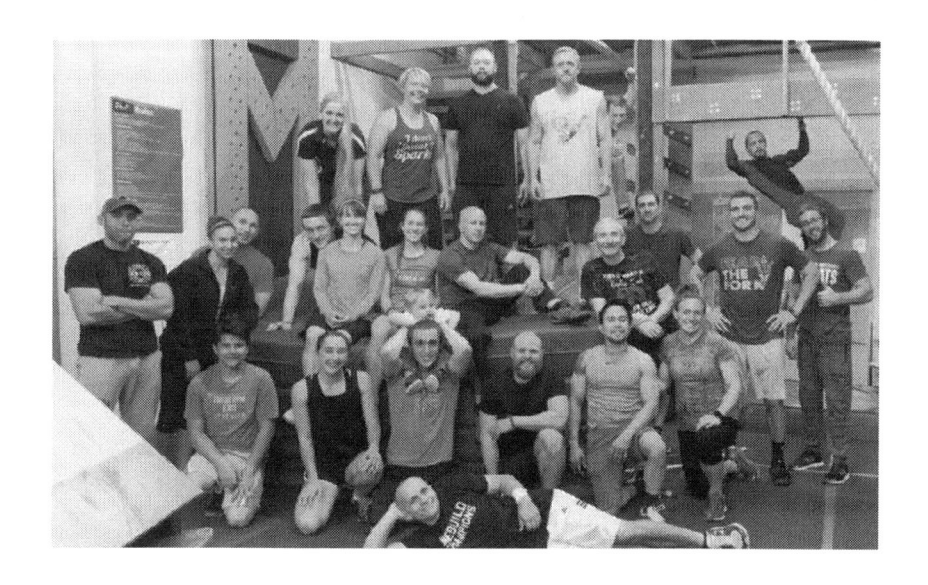

Walk-Ons Join the MLAB OH Mini-Comp

On Friday and Saturday, April 22nd and 23rd, Carolyn and I spent 24 hours in Chagrin Falls, near Cleveland, visiting our son,

Tim; his wife, Bonnie; our granddaughter Hannah; and our slightly-over-one-month-old granddaughter Lydia.

We headed home in time to allow me to participate in a mini-competition at Michelle's gym Saturday evening. I had not competed in quite some time, and I really wanted to participate in this one. We arrived home just in time for a quick bite before I headed to the gym.

When I got there I discovered that the already-formed Cleveland *ANW* walk-on line had decided to come down to Columbus to participate in the competition. They came to train and stay competition-sharp, so it was a fun competition.

As we were waiting in the hallway while the course was being set up behind closed doors, I asked questions about how the walk-on line worked, such as where were they meeting, where were they staying, and many other questions about the basics. It was all new to me.

You Should Join Them!

Some of my closer ninja friends heard me ask these questions. Immediately I heard, "You should go join them! That would be so cool! You should go do it!" With the encouragement of my peers and what I was learning about the line, a new door of consideration began to open in my mind.

I thought, "If I'm stuck in downtown Cleveland day after day, with check-in times for the line of 11:00 a.m. and 5:00 p.m., it could be a tremendous opportunity to work on *The Heart of a*

Ninja. It would be dedicated time each day at a local Panera, just writing and editing. Maybe this could be good."

When I mentioned this potential benefit out loud, the seed for this book surfaced. Shanon Paglieri said, "Your walk-on-line experience could be a great additional chapter for your book." Now my mind was really getting clouded with these possibilities influencing my potential decision.

I did okay in the mini-competition, completing five of the obstacles. As usual I went down earlier than I wanted to, but it was fun. I enjoyed interacting with the other competitors, who this time included the Cleveland walk-ons. And the walk-on-line option continued to marinate in the back of my mind.

Cheer, Test, or Walk-On

With the encouragement of my friends I felt like I should do a deep-dive assessment of my options. I had three options clearly in my mind. I could just go to Cleveland and cheer on Michelle and many other ninja friends. I could see if I could be a course tester, which might give me a chance to be on at least part of the course. Being a tester is no guarantee that you will be on an obstacle. *ANW* tries to get every tester on at least one obstacle, but it doesn't always work out. Or I could be a walk-on and hope to get a chance to run the course.

I decided what I really needed was a few blank pieces of paper and a pen. I took a few hours early that Sunday morning and sat down in the living room to pour through these options. I wanted to look at them holistically from many different perspectives:

What could happen if I...? What opportunities would come with each option? I listed the pros and cons of each option and set up a "decision tree" to be sure I made choices in the most logical order. I asked myself, "What could or would I get from each of these options and what could or would it cost for each of them?" The benefits of joining the walk-on line were surprisingly more than I had expected.

I also listed factors that needed to be considered in making this decision, including prior commitments that might be compromised if I went to Cleveland early to either test or be a walk-on. As I worked through these factors and commitments, time and money were significant considerations. I outlined a budget that I would need to consider if I were a tester or in the walk-on line. Since we had already planned to go to Cleveland as fans, I did not need to factor in the cost for the trip.

I did have several commitments over the next two-and-a-half weeks, but most of them could be rescheduled. There were two sessions with coaching clients I would need to reschedule, or I could meet with them by phone rather than in person. (Later in the week I reached out to each of them and they both gladly agreed to reschedule their coaching sessions to support my endeavor. They were both big fans of the show, of me, and of my ninja training activities.)

The decision tree revealed that if I wanted to join the walk-on line, time was of the essence. I would have days or weeks to decide between being a tester or just being a fan, but a decision to get in line needed to be made in the next day or so. This factor started to work on my mind... if I wanted the walk-on line to be an option I had to take action very soon.

The line had already been in existence for almost nine days. How badly did I want this to be an option? That was an important question, and I didn't have the answer. Another option popped up: solidify a spot (number) while I evaluated and considered staying in line for the duration; I could leave the line at any time but I could not put off joining the line and get an acceptably low number. At this point there were already nine in line. The next person to arrive would be number 10.

Let's Go for a Walk

I was able to focus on God pretty well during our church service that day, with only a little ninja warrior distraction. After church and lunch, Carolyn and I went for a walk, as it was a nice sunny day. It was a standard casual walk like we have enjoyed many times before, but when we started talking about ninja warrior I could hardly believe what was coming out of my mouth. I told Carolyn that I was toying with the idea that if I wanted the walk-on line to be an option I would need to head to Cleveland and get in line soon – as early as in the morning. Saying this to Carolyn out loud really surprised me. I had considered this option on paper but now I was stating it out loud, so I must have been thinking about it pretty seriously – much more seriously than I had realized.

Even after assessing my options that morning I had not landed on my decision, though I had determined that first I had to decide about the walk-on line, then decide about being a tester, and finally land at the default: cheering and being a fan, which would happen no matter what choice I made. The walk-on-line question had moved to the forefront of my mind.

Michelle's Dad

Based on a conversation I had had with Michelle the night before, I now felt that being Michelle's dad might limit my odds of running on the course rather than augment them. NBC features Michelle quite a lot. Maybe having her dad on the show as well would be just too much of a "Michelle" story. The senior casting producer had said as much a few months earlier. I tried to process this perspective, and it made sense in some ways, but it didn't make sense based on the feedback I had continually gotten from family, friends, and acquaintances.

NBC clearly knows who I am. They often refer to me and show me on the sidelines. It seemed to me and so many others that NBC would surely want to show the dad who had been featured so many times as a strong supporter on the sidelines now actually run the course. For the two years since I had completed an application and sent in a quality video, one of the *ANW* producers had made comments that he thought I would be "a shoe-in – a definite invitee." So since NBC still had not invited me, perhaps the Michelle factor really was at play.

If I chose to get in the walk-on line, I might be forcing the producers to take a harder stance if they did not want me to run. I could go through the walk-on-line experience and still be skipped even if I got in line early and received a low number. If I was going to do this, I had to be willing to go through the experience solely for the sake of the experience; it would not guarantee that I would get to run.

After a great deal of consideration I decided I was willing to do it just for the experience: getting to meet other ninjas, seeing what it is like to be in the walk-on line, and only *possibly* getting a chance to run. I worked hard to stay in this mindset; getting to run the course would simply be icing on the cake.

Lock In Now While I Can

Based on Carolyn's mild yet supportive response, I went to the Facebook Messenger thread that had been set up for those planning to go to Cleveland as competitors, testers, and fans and asked, "How many are currently in the walk-on line?" Immediately I received a flood of responses. Michelle said, "If you are considering joining the line, Dad, go now!" A bunch of others chimed in, "Go now! You should do it!" These responses messed up my head big time. I was considering leaving for Cleveland in the morning and joining the 11:00 a.m. check-in. What was all this "Go now!" stuff? "What's the big deal?" I asked myself.

As I continued to read the string, I learned quickly that the unofficial "pre-walk-on-line" runner order was based on when you arrived at the Great Lakes Science Center downtown. You had to take a photo of yourself and post it to the walk-on-line group chat to document your official arrival. It was like a postmark for mail. It was the date stamp for your arrival in the line.

Your place in line was not based on a formal 11:00 a.m. or 5:00 p.m. check-in time as I had thought.

I quickly learned that three other ninjas were on their way to join the line. My friends wanted me to leave right then so I could lock in at the number 10 spot. If I could get there next I would be runner number 10.

In the four prior 2017 *ANW* city qualifiers, about 17 walk-on-line ninjas got to compete per site. If this held true for Cleveland, leaving right then could put me in a strategic position. If I waited until morning I could be as high as number 13 or 14.

I left my computer to go find Carolyn. I shared with her the comments on Facebook and said, "I think I want to go, and now, to see if I can solidify a low number in the line, and while I'm in line I can decide if I want to stay or not." She responded, "Okay, if you *really* want to do this."

Fifteen-Minute Pack

I quickly headed upstairs and grabbed a few days' worth of clothes, then headed downstairs and grabbed some snacks, some reading material, a couple of CDs for my drives, plenty of notepaper and pens, a cooler, some drinks, and a few other things. I made sure I had a few hats, various layers of hoodies, and a coat.

Within 15 minutes I was on my way, driving to Cleveland to see what would happen, since I really didn't know how the walk-on line worked. Just before I left I posted on Facebook Messenger, "I'm on my way!"

With this fun "race" to Cleveland, with several ninjas on the road at the same time trying to get there first, a critical factor was to rein in my excitement and drive the speed limit. And being 60, I had to stop at rest areas more often than my younger peers, so I would likely get to Cleveland later than some of my peers might think. But I was on the road. Here we go! This new adventure had begun.

Add a Cold

Unfortunately I had come down with a mild cold. It started just after playing outside with my granddaughter Hannah in Tim and Bonnie's backyard. It had been warm at home, and I had expected the same weather at their house, but I was wrong. It was a lot cooler and I had brought only my red MLAB OH hoodie. I really should have worn a coat to play outside with Hannah, but you have to play with your granddaughter when you're in town, right? There is no other option. As always, it was so much fun.

When we returned home late that afternoon I could tell I had the front end of a cold. Regardless, I was on my way to Cleveland. I was going to give it a shot!

Chapter 4

Joining the Walk-On Line

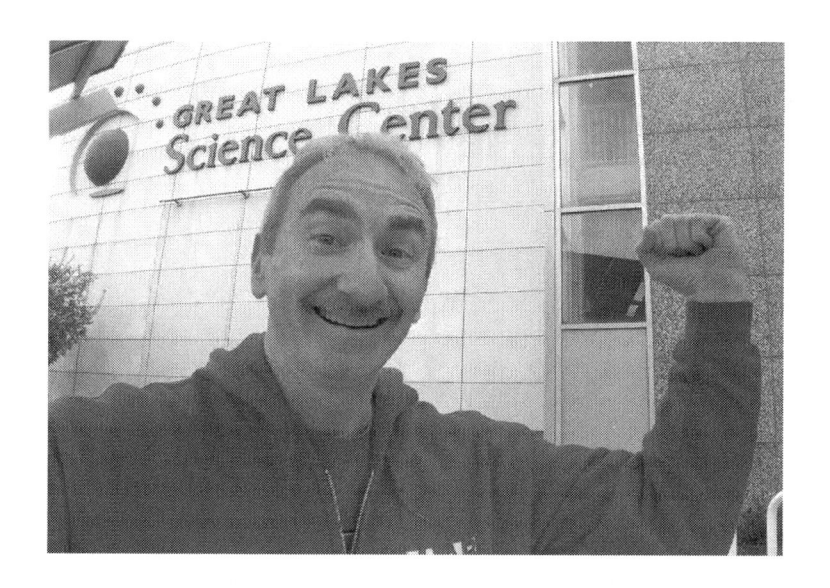

I'm Here! I'm Number 10! Now What?

It was Sunday night and I was in downtown Cleveland. There was not much activity in the area. It was 6:30 and the sun had not yet set. I thought I was in the right place. Did I need to park?

If so, where? What had Jesse said I needed to do? Take a picture documenting that I was there at that time?

My friends had said that time was of the essence. I jumped out of the car in the drop-off lane at the venue, the Great Lakes Science Center. My heart was pounding. I pulled out my phone, flipped up the camera screen to take a selfie, and positioned myself so that the camera could see me with the Science Center sign in the background. Snap! Woooo! It was done, whatever that meant or would mean. That photo was a lot more important than I dreamed.

Other ninjas were still on the road. I quickly looked up Facebook Messenger and the "Official Cleveland Standby Line" chat. I saw that Jesse had said I needed to take a photo in front of the firemen sculpture. Did I need to do that too or would the photo in front of the Science Center sign be good enough? I hoped it was good enough, and I had not yet seen the sculpture. (It was just a couple hundred feet ahead of me near the end of the Science Center drive loop.)

On the Messenger string I could see that ninjas were posting back and forth. "Where is he?" asked one ninja. Jesse was taking good care of me. "He's coming. He'll be here soon. He should be about 20 minutes away." I saw several other messages in the growing string as additional ninjas continued to join our special walk-on-line chat.

I selected the "add photo" option in Messenger, selected my brand new Science Center selfie, and hit "Enter." Wow! Another step complete. I figured I was now officially acknowledged and "in line," but how would I know?

Number 10

Soon a tall lanky guy with a brown journal in his hand approached my car with a grin. It was ninja Julien McConnell from the walk-on line. I recognized Julien both from seeing him in last year's walk-on line and from when the walk-ons had come to the MLAB OH mini-comp the night before. Things were happening so fast. He said, "You're in! You're number ten."

He opened his brown leather journal and flipped a few pages, and I saw the list of walk-on-line rules on the left-hand side. On the right I saw a list, and it produced a big smile on my face. I thought, "This really is it – this is happening!" He handed me his pen and on the next line I wrote "10" to the left, then printed my name to make sure others could read it; I had just driven over two hours to get there and I wasn't going to put this initial effort at risk with an illegible signature. I also filled in my phone number and the date I arrived.

I was the third person to sign in on Sunday the 23rd. Dan Galiczynski, number eight, and Brenda O'Hara, number nine, had signed in a little earlier. Brenda was the only woman in our line at that point.

I began to think, "Maybe I made the right choice to leave when I did." I thought I would have a pretty good chance to run if I was number 10. Ten was well within the range of those who had had a chance to run that year at other sites.

The first people on the list had signed in five days earlier on April 18th. Some of the guys had come the day after Easter. It wasn't until the next day that they decided to officially start the unofficial yet legitimate walk-on line.

On the list ahead of me were #1, Michael Nowoslawski; #2, Tyler Cravens; #3, Julien McConnell; #4, Jesse Wildman; #5, Rex Alba; #6, Danny Adair; #7, Noel Reyes; #8, Dan Galiczynski; and #9, Brenda O'Hara.

As I mentioned earlier, Jesse is a friend and an MLAB OH instructor. I had spent many hours training with Jesse at our gym and I had learned a lot from this strong and growing ninja. He is quite an athlete.

Columbus ninja Rex Alba was also in line ahead of me. I had trained on and off with Rex over the past four years. He's one of the ninjas who participated in competitions Michelle had hosted at the climbing gym Vertical Adventures before she opened MLAB OH. On occasion Rex would show up at MLAB OH so I had gotten to know him much better, though he was not a regular. Since that time Rex has become a good ninja friend and a member of our Lunch Time Training Partners (LTTPs) at MLAB OH. He has been such an encouragement and inspiration as he has continued to get so much stronger as a ninja.

More ninjas came during the next 24 hours, just as I had been told they would on the Messenger string. Three more Ninjas came before daybreak the next morning: Jonathan Angelilli got there at 9:43 p.m., a little over three hours after I arrived. He had come from New York. From Michigan, Tommy Daly arrived and checked in at 12:28 a.m., very early Monday morning. That was just six hours after me. Joshua Sanchez, driving through the night, had also come from the East Coast and arrived at 4:29 a.m.

As you can see, everyone was really dedicated to this effort. Steve Leppo was the next ninja to arrive. He got there the next day in time for our 11:00 a.m. check-in on Tuesday, April 25th, and was number 14.

The Walk-On-Line Rules

The rules for the walk-on line were simple and seemed logical to me. They were: No posting on public social media about the line or about being in line (only on the exclusive Facebook Messenger feed); check in every day at 11:00 a.m. and 5:00 p.m. at the corner of the Cleveland Browns Stadium just across from the Great Lakes Science Center; if you miss one check-in you get bumped back one spot in the line; if you miss two check-ins you get bumped to the back of the line; there is a 15-minute buffer on the check-in time. Short and simple. The rules were easy to understand and follow if you were truly dedicated. I appreciated the structure. Thanks Julien, or whoever came up with them.

We continued to use Facebook Messenger to communicate updates and joke around with each other outside of our official check-in times. Several ninjas thought it would be fun to change their names on the Facebook string. They changed them to names like Goldie Locks and Waldo 2. They were just having fun, but for this 60-year-old it got very confusing who was saying what.

The Golden Ticket

On Monday our number-one ninja in line, Michael Nowoslawski, had a scheduled TV interview with the local NBC affiliate. We were joking and wishing that maybe at the end of the interview he would get invited to compete on *ANW*. As you can imagine, when you're waiting in line you can come up with all kinds of possibilities that could work to your benefit, individually or as a group.

That evening we conducted our check-in a little early and concluded it quickly to allow Michael and a few guys who were good friends to head to his house for that interview. I didn't get a chance to see it, but Michael has a great ninja obstacle setup in his backyard, and that's where the local NBC affiliate wanted to conduct the interview, which had been arranged for some time but because of various conflicts did not happen until Michael had already been in the walk-on line for a few days.

In the early evening I saw on our Messenger string that Michael had been invited to compete on *ANW*. To his surprise, at the end of the interview he was presented with a Golden Ticket and was no longer a walk-on.

Our group was so excited for him. This also meant that all of us moved up one slot. It was a win-win for all of us. I was now number nine and my chance to run got even better. We were excited for Michael and for ourselves.

I personally know of at least three cases when ninjas were in a walk-on line for one city and got invited to compete in another city. I'm sure there have been many more cases like this. You never know what's going to happen.

More Ninjas Join the Line

Two additional ninja friends joined the line during the next week. Scott Walberry came on Thursday evening and Bryce LaRoche joined on Friday. Both guys are great ninja athletes. Scott is so impressive, especially for being 51 years old. You would never know it. Scott signed in on line 15 of our book, which placed him as our 14th line member, right after Steve Leppo.

Bryce is one of my favorite ninjas to watch compete. He has not yet been on the show but I've seen him in many local competitions. A quiet guy, he is so skilled and strong. He has won many of the competitions in which I've competed. I was pumped that he was joining us. He joined as number 16 on the official Julien book, placing him as number 15 with the exit of Michael.

There were two ninjas who had not yet competed on the show that I really wanted to see run in 2018: Sean Noel and Bryce LaRoche. Sean did get a late call to compete, which was so exciting. At the time he was an instructor at MLAB OH. He has shared so many great tips with Central Ohio ninjas, and always demonstrated how a technique should look. He is such a great athlete and I really wanted to see what he could do on the *ANW* course.

The other was Bryce, as I mentioned — now effectively number 15 in our line, which gave him a pretty good chance to run —

never a guarantee, but a very good chance. This was going to be a very fun year, especially if I got to see those two run the course.

Steve Leppo and Scott Walberry had work commitments they were trying to manage while they were in line. At one point Steve had to miss a check-in due to work. He knew it would cost him one place in line, but he had to do it for his job. He moved back to number 14 and Scott moved into slot number 13.

A few days later Scott also had to miss a check-in time. He reasoned that this would simply put him back in his original slot of 14. As it worked out Steve had the opportunity to run the course and Scott did not. I think both guys felt like they did the right thing and what they needed to do for their jobs. It was a shame that one of them got to run and the other did not. They both knew it was a risk, and that's the way *ANW* works.

So Close, but No

As I shared earlier, NBC usually runs walk-ons three times during the night — at the very beginning of the night, immediately following the crew lunch break at midnight or 1:00 a.m., and at the end of the night if they have run all the invited ninjas and it's still dark. Once there's light on the horizon, they stop filming. NBC loves the glamour and glitz of the night-time scene with the lights flashing all around the course.

During this qualifier night a ninja was injured, a broken obstacle had to be fixed, and there were slightly more finishers than at some other qualifiers. These all took time and reduced the number of walk-ons who got to compete in Cleveland.

NBC used 10 walk-ons at the beginning of the night. After the crew lunch break two additional walk-ons got to run. Scott Walberry would have been next, at about 1:00 a.m. They pulled him up onto the stage to get ready to run, then he was pulled back down when the producers changed their minds.

He had one more hope. He would be the first walk-on at the end of the night if there was still time. Had there been even five more minutes of darkness he would likely have competed. He was so close, twice, but he did not get the chance to run.

He was probably pretty frustrated. You know when you get in the walk-on line that there is no guarantee you will get to run, but you hope with your entire being that it will work out. You hope you made a good investment of your time, money, and sacrifice.

After Scott got through the initial shock of not running and had time to reflect on his experience, he shared a powerful Facebook post. It reflected a great-big-picture perspective. I asked him for permission to share it here, and he agreed.

Scott Walberry May 10 at 9:23pm · Cleveland, OH ·

> Glad to be home from an interesting journey. One of the things I'm trying to do in my desire toward personal growth is to reflect and be grateful. Sometimes gratitude is not as easy as it seems, but being denied an opportunity to play on a glorified jungle gym for adults is nothing compared to the adversity so many others are experiencing.

Early Tuesday morning, I must admit I was feeling bitter, discouraged, angry, dejected, etc. about missing my opportunity that I've passionately pursued for well over a year by ONE spot.

I had spot number 13, and was told up front that there are no guarantees for any walk-ons, but time permitting, the producer will do his best to get us on.

The first 10 went right away, which included two of my training partners from the gym which was great to see. A couple of unfortunate injuries and an obstacle malfunction led to some delays that put the schedule behind. Around 1 am, the crew's lunch break was announced despite being about 10-15 runners behind schedule. During that lunch break, walk ons 11-15 were told to warm up and be ready, which we did. Keep in mind we had to be there at 5 pm, so this was 7 hours of checking in and just waiting for the announcement to report to the starting area.

Walk on #11 leads off, just two away until my big shot. WO #12, I'm on deck. As I'm getting mentally prepared for the first obstacle, the producer is told to bump me due to the schedule being behind, they need to resume with the competitors who were called. I had a feeling right then that I may not get back to that spot. As the moon was descending toward the west, I knew before long that the sun would be unable to be stopped rising to the east. With about three runners to go around 5:45 am, light started to appear as the last runner made his way through the course. The producer called us together to announce what I was fearing more than any obstacle on the course. "This is it." The truth is, although I was freezing; mentally, emotionally, and physically exhausted, I wasn't nearly as prepared as I had been five hours earlier, yet it still was devastating to hear those three words. The venue emptied in no time, and as I walked the three blocks, toward the hotel, I began thinking about the time and money wasted pursuing this. "Maybe I should just give up... I just want to drive home." Just a bunch of negative garbage thinking. Why me? Then I remembered something I read in the book The Noticer by Andy Andrews. Instead of saying Why me?, how about trying a different perspective, "Why not me?"

I can embrace being the first person not to run. In fact, that can be the theme for next year's submission video. Only five other people in the country will share the title with me as "The first person in the walk-on line not to run." Now that is elite company.

This story is not over, in fact it has just begun. Stay tuned.

Thanks, Scott, for being who you are and being an encouragement and light to us all. This was a tough challenge and you came through it better, not bitter. You will have a better future because of your perspective and the choices you have made.

Bryce did not get to run either. In addition, there were 15 other ninjas who came to the walk-on line over those last 10 days who also did not get a chance to run. I felt especially sorry for these two good friends, Scott and Bryce.

What was it like to effectively live out of town in downtown Cleveland for over two weeks? In the next chapter I share many of my initial experiences being in downtown Cleveland while in the walk-on line.

Chapter 5

Being in Downtown Cleveland

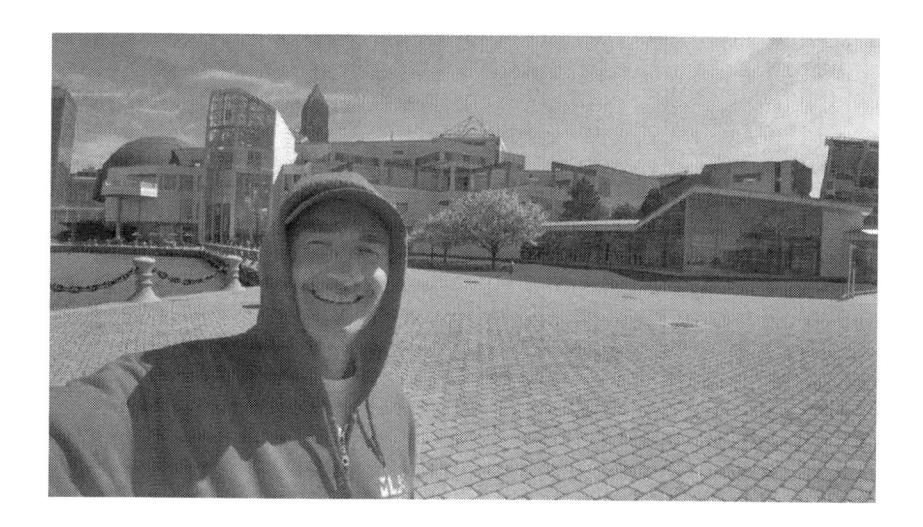

I don't go to a downtown very often, so I don't think in terms of parking costs. I received a rude awakening, or reality check, that most parking in large city downtowns is paid parking. Parking is at a premium, so they charge for it. With my quick bolt from our house on Sunday afternoon, I was not prepared for parking meters. There were many available meters by our check-in area, and there were all-day parking lots available, but I wasn't sure I was going to stay downtown all day; I didn't know how I was going to use my time. The check-in requirement gave us about five-and-a-half hours to use in some way each day we were there. It was critical to check in at 5:00 p.m. Even one miss or late appearance would cause me to get bumped a spot in line.

At home I normally drive once or twice a day and only four to six miles – about 15 minutes' driving spread throughout my day. I drive to MLAB OH, to the local Panera, or maybe to Lowes or another store. All of these are about two miles away. Other than major trips, over the past five years I normally drove my car about 2,000 miles a year, so I clearly don't drive very much. I have been very happy with this routine. Even the drive to our church once a week is only about five miles.

Spending all those days in downtown Cleveland was going to be a big change – not a problem, just a big shift. I was also sensitive about the impact this "little adventure" would have on our family budget. It had not been budgeted, and we have lived by a budget now for over 39 years, which is one of the key reasons I was able to retire at age 56.

That Sunday morning I had calculated the worst-case scenario for out-of-pocket expenses. Based on my projections it could cost up to $750 to participate in the walk-on line, if it took the full 16 days and if I elected to drive all the way home each day. This option was not my first choice, but it was an option; it would have cost much more if I had stayed at a hotel each night. I ended up staying at Tim's home in Chagrin Falls, a Cleveland suburb, for many of the nights.

Parking

The all-day parking lots charged $5 or $6 a day. At 16 days, that alone would cost $80 to $100. With this option I would also need to find a place to go and something to do from 11:00 to 5:00 every day. And I would have to eat downtown, likely at a greater cost than if I left the downtown area.

So I elected to use parking meters near the check-in location. They required 25¢ for a short period of time, usually 15 minutes. I didn't have any quarters in my car, but soon I found myself stockpiling quarters in the cubbyholes of my car dashboard. I intentionally bought most of my meals with cash, strategizing for more change, quarters in particular. The meters took both dimes and nickels, but the best value was with quarters.

For most check-ins I would arrive at least 20 minutes early. None of us wanted to risk missing a check-in because of some surprise traffic issue or accident along our path. Jesse was usually there first, just before me. Later on Bryce was also one of the early arrivers. For our morning check-ins he would often drive from home, which was a couple of hours away.

I was happy to find a coin dispenser by the restrooms in the Great Lakes Science Center basement. It provided quarters from bills for those wanting to buy food or drinks from the vending machines. The first time I discovered this machine I loaded up with five dollars of quarters. I was set to go for at least the next several days.

To save on costs, a number of us would sit in our cars until close to the check-in time and only put quarters in to cover the time we would be away from our cars, which could be 15 to 30 minutes. We'd go through our formal check-in process, share any key updates, coordinate activities for the day, and joke around. The joking happened a lot and added to the experience for us all as we grew closer and closer as a walk-on family.

Several times Bryce and I had peculiar experiences feeding the parking meters. I got a kick out of them – more of a kick than Bryce. Once, even though we were using meters that shared the same post, my quarter provided me with 20 minutes and Bryce got the standard 15 minutes. Another time, later that same day, we shared meter posts again at another spot along that street. Bryce was excited to get 20 minutes for his quarter, but I got 30 minutes. I just told him, "I have the touch." We joked about me putting his quarters in the meter for him. We didn't test this concept, but it was another fun memory for this crazy walk-on-line experience.

Bathrooms

Something else that I was not accustomed to was having to search for a bathroom. This is where the Great Lakes Science Center really came into play. They had a nice public bathroom on the bottom level of the facility. Due to the time it took me to drive there, I often needed a restroom right after I arrived. It became a routine for some of us to get parked with a little time before the check-in and walk to the Science Center restroom. This was a life-saver; it was much more critical for me, at age 60, than for many of the others in our line.

The Check-In Process

The check-in process was simple for this unofficial trust-based group. Once we arrived, Julien would pull out his little brown book and flip open to the list of names. He would read each name with his own flair and name enhancements, and we would respond indicating we were there. You could hear a quiet or bold "Here," "Yo," "Present," "Yah Man," "Yah Dude," "Yup," and many others' "I am here" statements. It took only about a minute to go through this short list. Then we received any updates that Julien or others had heard about our process and timing with *ANW*. We would also ask who was doing what that day or night. There were times when the whole gang coordinated to do something together. Most of the time we broke into smaller groups or just made our own plans for how to spend the in-between time.

I had hoped to write much more of *The Heart of a Ninja* in between check-ins. I did get some writing time in, but not as much as I expected. I just did not feel like writing due to my cold, not having a good place to write, and just wanting to spend time with the other ninjas to hang out, mini-train, or whatever. They were becoming my new family.

The last element of our check-in process was confirming the next check-in time. A few times we adjusted the time slightly or picked a different check-in place, and once, with everyone's agreement, we canceled a check-in.

Our Growing Gang

Our gang grew to 19 ninjas the night before the official *ANW* walk-on-line start time, which was Wednesday, May 3rd, at 10:00 a.m. Our number jumped to 29 over those last few hours.

Just a few days before the competition one of our low-number walk-ons was required by *ANW* to leave the line. We were very sorry to hear about the situation. It would have been so much fun to see him run, but it was not to be, at least for that qualifier. This change resulted in most of us moving down again by one number. I became number eight. Wow! It was feeling more and more likely that I would get a chance to run!

For me there was always the question of what to do for dinner. Should I leave downtown immediately following our 5:00 p.m. check-in and join thousands of other drivers heading home, or find a place to hang out for an hour or two and let the traffic die down? I used both strategies. Sometimes I went for a walk to the Great Lakes Science Center and the waterfront, walked around the Browns' stadium, or explored the downtown streets through the tall buildings. Sometimes I took a short drive in heavy traffic to a fast-food restaurant. There I could order dinner and either read or write for 60 to 90 minutes while the traffic was ebbing. Even this option took a good deal of time and patience because it could take 15 to 20 minutes to go just six or eight blocks to a Burger King or a McDonald's. Other times I would bite the bullet, join the rest of the traffic, and make my way out of town toward Chagrin Falls where Tim's family lives.

Once I was within a few miles of Tim's house I would visit a pizza or sub shop for 60 to 90 minutes. My goal was to not arrive at their home earlier than 8:30 p.m. so that I would not disrupt my granddaughter's bedtime routine. Her grandfather (me) can get her worked up pretty quickly, which can lead to a challenging "go to bed" experience for the family. Arriving after 8:30 prevented such disruptions.

When I was still dealing with my cold, which had gotten worse, a few times I grabbed a quick bite at a fast-food restaurant and drove to a grocery store parking lot close to Tim's home. There I tried to sleep in the car until my phone alarm rang and get to Tim's house just a little after 8:30.

My Cold Got Worse

Since the year 2000 my core gets cold much more quickly than it used to. Based on my doctor's challenge to me that year, I changed my lifestyle, which significantly improved my cholesterol level. I also lost 30 pounds. These were great changes – just what the doctor ordered.

I started exercising daily, primarily on the treadmill. I cut down on French-fry consumption. I scaled back on ice cream, limiting my portions using a little kitchen scale. I now dish out only two or three ounces of low-fat ice cream. I also stopped putting butter or margarine on anything – and I mean anything! I still eat foods that have butter in them; I just don't add butter on top. If I feel the need to add something to my bread, potatoes, or vegetables, I use a little olive oil. I no longer put butter on toast, waffles, English muffins, pancakes, potatoes, bread, or anything. Nothing! I've been living this more healthy lifestyle for over 18 years. But since that initial weight loss (I have put some of it back on over the years, but some of that is new muscle from all of my ninja training), I get colder; I don't have enough fat to keep me warm.

That Saturday morning with my granddaughter when I didn't have a coat, my core felt cold, and that feeling often is followed by a runny nose, some congestion, and/or a sore throat. All of these started that afternoon just before we left for home and lingered for the next few days as I started living through this walk-on-line experience. On day three in the line my cold took a much deeper dive. I was miserable! If I had been home I would have been in bed for two or three days trying to recover. But that was not an option. I had to show up for each check-in time and find a way to use my time while nursing myself back to health. All of this was taking place while I spent time with a bunch of great ninjas who constantly wanted to play, train, and exercise.

My car became my personal hospital room. I stocked it with Kleenex and a ton of cough drops, and day by day I added to my medications since I was not getting any better. I bought Vicks Nyquil, Dayquil, and VapoRub. I purchased a nose spray, and I even bought some 24-hour allergy pills to see if they would help. I bought a gallon of orange juice that I consumed over a four-day period. I tried not to overlap these medications, but I did try and/or use most of them during a five-day period in line. It was ugly and a real pain. It really took a toll on my body, which was supposed to be getting ready to run an *ANW* course in a few days. You do what you can with what you have, so I just kept pushing through during this hard time. I rested a lot, either reclined in my driver's seat or lying on the ground in the park. I needed rest and I tried my best to get it.

Some of these days were rainy, which made this experience even more ugly. It was clearly not my favorite situation: sick, rainy, stuck in a car, having to drive in a downtown environment. The flip side was that I had the opportunity to be around an amazing group of healthy, bouncing-off-the-walls ninjas. This added to my very memorable walk-on-line experience.

The Facebook Messenger Thread

These ninjas were all younger than I, and many of them by more than 25 years. I am over twice the age of most of them, but we still related well in so many ways.

One way that was a little difficult for me was the way Facebook Messenger was used. For many of them it's a fun tool for joking conversations, short statements, and GIFs (videos). They had a ball going back and forth multiple times within a minute.

At my age, being retired and oriented toward a budget (which I manage judiciously to limit expenses), all I could think about was my cell phone data costs. I wasn't on WiFi and had to use data in downtown Cleveland. I normally leave data turned off on my phone and turn it on only when I want to get an update. I find this works pretty well, and it helped me reduce my data needs by over two gig a month. I went from using over 2.5 gig a month to often being under .5 gig. Carolyn, Michelle, and I shared a plan, and this reduction allowed us to stay on a 6-gig plan, saving us a lot of money that I would rather spend on fun ninja competition trips.

The ninjas were having a blast, back and forth with GIF after GIF after GIF. In my head all I could think was "data, data, data." Carolyn helped me discover that my phone had been set up to automatically save photos and videos that came in through Facebook Messenger. I was apparently blowing through data even more than I thought. She found that I had used 1.1 gig of data in only four days in Cleveland. That was over twice what I would use for a full month at home.

I viewed Messenger as a place to get important walk-on-line updates, and all the GIFs made it hard to find them. For many of the young ninjas who were actively engaged in the banter, getting key information was not that big of a deal because they were reading and reacting to every post that appeared; they weren't going to miss anything.

I was fearful I would miss something important that could be sandwiched in the middle of 30 or 40 GIFs. I was trying not to turn my data on and see all the conversation and GIFs. I just wanted to see information updates: time changes, location changes, new information about the arrival of the senior casting producer, etc. The number of GIFs was fine but I was distracted by them.

We come from different generations with different types of fun. I tried to appreciate our differences, as I'm older and have different priorities and perspectives, and I was glad they were having fun and bonding through this activity. I made it through, maybe not quite as easily as many of the others, but I didn't miss any key information – I was just afraid that I would.

I wondered if they had unlimited data plans and what that cost. It was probably not that big of a deal for them. Being retired and living on your investments can change your outlook on expenses.

Some of the language and content were different from what I'm normally exposed to as well. I dealt with these differences for this short window of time.

Trashed Car

I don't keep my car as clean as Carolyn keeps hers. I keep a variety of things in my front and back seats and my trunk that I might need: scrap paper, pens, CDs, a little pillow, an exercise ball, an exercise band, and several little items for traveling; not to mention the balance obstacles I keep in the trunk for when I have a chance to use them.

Nearly living in my car with a cold for two weeks took my amount of stuff and messiness to a whole new level. I had a water bottle; a little cooler; orange juice; cough drops, nasal spray, and all those medicines I mentioned above; a book as a writing surface for when I made notes; old drink bottles; a zip-lock bag filled with quarters – and so much more. I tried to have most of these within reach when I was driving. It really got messy, even for my relaxed standards of what you should keep in a car.

It was no longer a car; it was a version of a hotel room where I needed whatever it took to live between about 9:30 a.m. and nearly 8:30 p.m. I spent many of these days and hours literally in my car. This was a whole new experience that I don't want to repeat in the future. I could have been more efficient, but with my cold I was in survival mode for much of that time.

I used Kleenex and cough drops like they were water, blowing or dabbing my runny nose with the tissues and continually sucking on the cough drops. I visited the store several times to get new supplies for the car and my hoodie pockets. It was a rough time.

I continually said to myself, "Just make it through another few hours until the next check-in. Then you can drive back to Tim's and get some rest before you get up to do it all again, hopefully a little stronger tomorrow." I would then tag on, "And yes, some sunshine tomorrow would really be great." We did have some sunshine during those walk-on days but we had our share of rain and drizzle as well. I'm sure having a cold made more of my days feel gloomy.

Where do you go when you're confined for hours a day out of town for two weeks? You will read how I solved this challenge in the next chapter.

Chapter 6

Finding a Place to Be

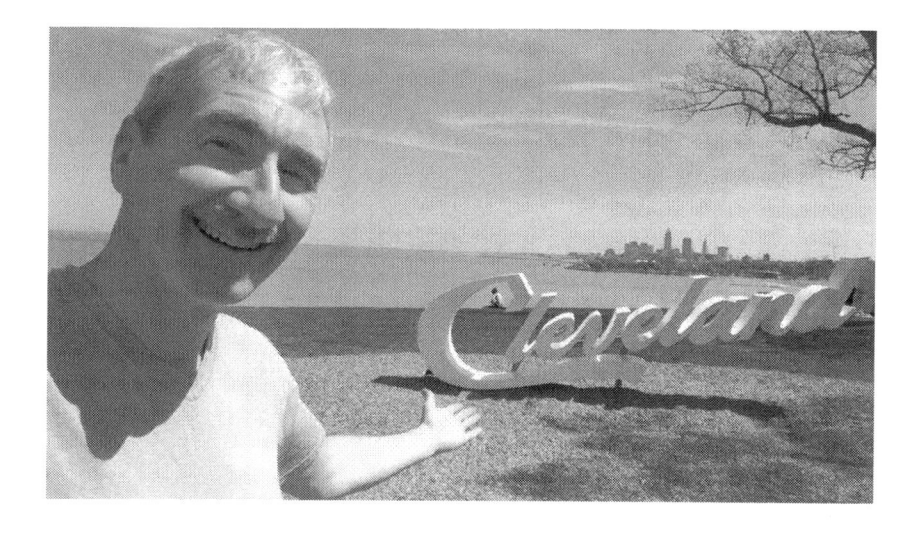

I am a very comfortable guy living in a paid-off home and not having to spend additional money just to be somewhere. It was a good experience to see how awkward or hard it can be when you don't have a home or a place to stay, be, or spend time.

It cost money to keep me or my car just about anywhere. If I wanted to be somewhere to read, to write *The Heart of a Ninja*, to think, or to sleep, I had to spend money to park, or pay (make a purchase) to be there. I bought several meals, often fast food, at off hours when the restaurants were not very busy so that I wouldn't feel rushed or feel the need to leave. After two to four hours of slowly eating my meal and refreshing my soft drink several times, I would eventually leave. There were a few times when I felt guilty about loitering after an hour or so, so I would buy cookies or an ice cream sundae. This was "of course" to pay for my time at the restaurant. It had nothing to do with my sweet tooth.

It felt safe to spend the five or six hours between check-ins at these restaurants. They provided me with a place to do Well Done Life coaching-related work, write, or enjoy some reading. I did this the first few days; then I discovered Edgewater Park. There were no soft-drink dispensers at the park, which I'm sure was good for me.

I was writing *The Heart of a Ninja* at one of these restaurants when I saw a note on our Messenger string from one of our walk-on-line members. He was letting me know that some of the ninjas were going to a park to set up and play on a slack line. I was thankful for the heads-up. I replied, "Thanks. I'm at a fast-food restaurant writing more of my book. Thanks for letting me know." His quick reply was "Which restaurant?" I shared the name and location, and was surprised to see his quick response: "That's the same restaurant where Jesse was held up with a knife just a few days ago." This new information immediately put me on edge. It caused me to quickly glance around the restaurant and pay much better attention to my surroundings. I stayed there just a little longer, but not as long as I had planned. Safety first. Keeping my eyes alert to my surroundings, I quickly moved to my car, tossed my computer bag into the front seat, got in, closed the door, locked the doors, and put my seat belt on while I checked my rear view mirror. I then quickly backed out and pulled out of the parking lot onto the street, where I took a nice deep breath and began to feel my heart start to slow down again.

Later I learned that the holdup had occurred after dark when Jesse was walking back to his car. He was not hurt and only lost a little money. He was thankful he didn't have his wallet on him.

These were some of the eye-openers that I do not routinely experience in my comfortable suburban home. This was good – though not fun – exposure for me to better appreciate what I have and what some others deal with all the time. I'm very thankful for who I am and where I am in life.

Edgewater Park

Edgewater Park was my paradise during my time in Cleveland. It provided two very important services: free parking and public bathrooms. These were two of the most important criteria for my time between check-ins. Upper Edgewater Park is less than 10 minutes north, up the western coast of the lake. This short drive was very practical for getting back in time to our designated check-in place.

And it's a very nice park. It provides a great view of downtown Cleveland. In front of the downtown overlook there is a very nice "Cleveland" sign. Visitors repeatedly took photos in front of this sign. I did the same several times to help cement this experience in my mind for the rest of my life.

At one point, after some rain, there was a small break in the clouds and the sun shone right through that hole onto the Cleveland sign alone. It really made the sign pop! It didn't matter how badly I was feeling at that time, I had to get out and take one more picture of that sign with the cityscape of Cleveland in the background. It was so perfect – surreal.

The park had a nice grassy area where, when I was feeling up to it, I set up the balance obstacles I keep in my car. It also has trees a perfect distance from each other for setting up a slack line. A few times some of the other ninjas set up a slack line there. Because of my poor physical condition I normally just watched, sometimes lying down in the grass. I was just trying to get more rest.

Also at the park was a little shelter or pavilion intended to provide shade over a picnic table. It was made of iron, so hanging from it with our weight was not going to damage it. It was an artistic, three-sided structure that could be used as a great cliffhanger – a very difficult one – with a hard, sharp, iron edge. The side closest to the table tilted forward, which made it even harder to climb with just hands. I tried to climb across various portions of this structure and could only make it part way on any side.

I pointed out the structure to Bryce and Scott. Bryce went over to the iron structure, pulled himself up on the hardest side, and proceeded to move "hands only" around the whole structure, duplicating the hard side and finishing with a few pull-ups. We had some really strong ninjas in our line! Go Bryce!

The Library – A Great Quiet Place to Focus and Write

It wasn't till one of the last days I was in line that I located the Walz Branch of the Cleveland Public Library near Edgewater Park. During one of my quick return trips home Carolyn suggested I look for a library, and it was an ideal, quiet place to spend time – an excellent place to read or write. It would have been a great free option to have used earlier.

A Place to Sleep

Each of us faced the challenge of finding a place to sleep. We solved this challenge in many ways. Several walk-ons accepted Brenda O'Hara's offer to stay at her family home in a Cleveland suburb. They drove in with her each day. I heard they helped around the house and cooked meals for Brenda and her family. This was a win-win for all of them.

Michael Nowoslawski, our "Golden Ticket" number-one guy in line who ended up getting invited to compete, also housed a few ninjas. At least one guy stayed at a downtown hotel. A number of us either drove home each night – up to a couple of hours away – or stayed with family or friends in the area.

One guy, managing his limited resources, stayed in his van overnight in a paid parking lot for almost the entire time. Jonathan Angelilli from New York stayed with a friend and rode his bike into downtown for each of our check-ins.

I was able to stay with Tim and his family, who live about 30 miles southeast of downtown Cleveland. I stayed at his home eight nights. Twice I made the two-hour drive home at night and made the return trip in the morning for our 11:00 a.m. check-in. I left extra early from home on those days; I drive the speed limit and I wanted to make sure I had enough time even if construction or accidents got in my way.

It was great to stay with Tim and his family. They were very hospitable the entire time, providing a place for me to stay any night I needed it. As I mentioned, I was careful to ensure that I would arrive in the evening at a time that would not interfere with the sleep schedule of my three-year-old granddaughter, who loves to play with her grandpa. Most mornings I had a couple of hours to play with both her and her three-month-old sister before I left for downtown for our morning check-in. I really enjoyed the extra time with Tim and his family, and thank them so much for welcoming me into their home.

A lot happened as we waited and spent time in downtown Cleveland between our check-in times. In the next chapter you will read about the many planned and unplanned experiences.

Chapter 7

Cleveland Experiences

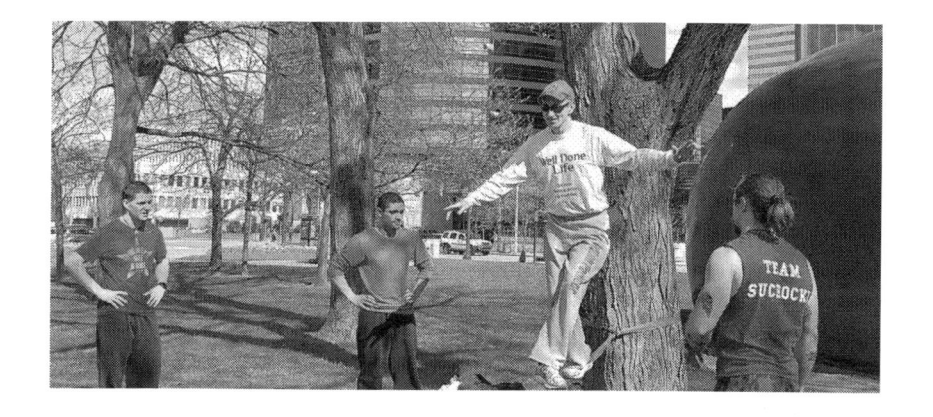

Mini-Training

With my limited physical condition and no access to MLAB OH, I came up with other ways to train. I felt like I should be doing something; I could be running the *ANW* course in just a few days!

I took advantage of my drive-time by regularly working with purple putty I had received from an occupational therapist. A few months earlier I had jammed the pinky on my left hand while attempting to catch an eight-foot lache (a swing between horizontal bars). Due to how badly I jammed it and how long it was taking to heal, I got a referral from my doctor to an occupational therapist who helped me exercise it. The therapist gave me the putty, which was a great tool not only for healing my pinky but for building strength in all my fingers. I used it each morning and evening during my 30- to 45-minute drive to and from downtown. Each trip I would squeeze the putty at least 20 times with each hand. As little as it seemed, at least I felt like I was doing something to maintain or build strength for a potential *ANW* run.

Michelle gave me a Flexbar Theraband, which is a rubber bar I use to address my tennis elbow. I used it to strengthen my grip, to roll on my thighs while driving, and as a back support during the drives.

I also did stretching and pulling exercises with my hands on my steering wheel. These came in handy, and I thank ninja friend and doctor, Peggy Hale, for suggesting them a few months earlier.

A few times I pulled my balance obstacles out of my trunk to practice on. I have a variety of PVC pipes cut to various lengths so I can practice walking across them in different ways: rolling forward, rolling left or right, standing upright, walking across the top, etc.

I also have a number of two-by-fours in various lengths and glued together in various ways that I practice walking across. These are very handy, but dangerous, as you will soon find out.

Getting to spend at least a little time on this training equipment helped me mentally. At least I was doing something during this very awkward time while I was sick and in the walk-on line.

The Bruise

As though having a cold wasn't bad enough, I faced an additional challenge. I was at Edgewater Park with Scott Walberry and Bryce LaRoche and we set up a few obstacles from my trunk in the grass to practice running across. I selected a few short four-inch PVC pipes, a few short two-by-four obstacles, and a few colorful half balls I had purchased. We set some of them sideways, some long-ways, and even upright, and in a variety of combinations, and had fun running through these little balance challenges.

On a number of occasions we went down and hit the soft grass, which worked quite well as a mat. I went down more than they did. It was great practice and a lot of fun. I like to switch things up, so I was continually changing the order or the direction of the obstacles. As we successfully made it through the lineup I would also increase the distance between some of the obstacles. It didn't take long for us to practice and master various setups; then I would make yet another change.

About 15 minutes into our play time I was making my way through one of the setups and came to where I had to step on top of a five-inch PVC pipe standing on its end. I had walked through this obstacle many times in the past – slowly, very slowly – but often successfully. This time as I put my weight on this obstacle, it tilted to the side. It might have been the grass or dirt giving way, though both Scott and Bryce had made it through this exact step, but it fell to the side, my feet went to the right, and I went down on my left hip and my hands, much as I had already done a few times that day.

This time was different! The very next obstacle was a set of glued-together two-by-fours standing upright about four inches high. It would have been my next step with my left foot, but there was no way my foot was going to get it this time. I did, however, fall directly on the center of the two-by-fours with my left hip. As I hit it with all my falling weight, my momentum forced the obstacle to fall over as I slid sideways with it. Ouch! Wow, did that sting! I could not hide the sharp pain that shot through my hip, though I thought it would just be a little bruise. I quickly rolled over onto my other side and worked to get to my knees so I could stand up and start to walk it off. Scott and Bryce quickly came to my rescue, asking if I was okay. I assured them I would be fine as I very slowly stood myself up and started to try and walk off the pain.

Wow! It was still really hurting. But I'm a ninja. I couldn't let this shut me down, especially in front of Scott and Bryce. I took a few steps and told them I was going to walk over to the bathroom, which was a good 50 yards away. Wow again. This was really stinging, and I was definitely hobbling as I slowly made my way over to the bathroom.

It hit me that we were now less than a week from potentially running on the *ANW* course. I was already fighting my bad cold. I was living in a very awkward environment in the walk-on line with ninjas who were more than 25 years younger than I. Scott, who was 51, was the only one close to my age. Now I was going to have to recover from this very painful injury that was keeping me from walking normally. I was quickly reminded that the first obstacle on *ANW* is the ascending steps that require you to use your hips to push off and throw your body left and right across each of the steps. All I could think about was what else could go wrong as I moved closer to getting to run on the course.

When I arrived at the bathroom I pulled down my sweatpants to see my left side. I knew from the pain that there was going to be a massive dark-blue bruise on my hip, but there was almost nothing – no sign at all of an injury. I couldn't believe it. Surely on the side of my hip would be some evidence of how hard I hit that two-by-four, but the answer was no – not much to show for all that pain.

I slowly hobbled back to my obstacles. By then Scott and Bryce had had enough work on them, and I was in no condition to attempt them again, so they helped me gather them up and take them to the car.

I was still stinging and very sore. I found it very hard to walk anywhere near normally. What would this mean if I did get a chance to run the course? After this ninjury I began to fear that if I did get to run the course I would really embarrass myself and my friends because I had become only a fraction of the ninja they had known. It was getting very scary.

My walking improved over the next several days. I wasn't going to spend any more time training, especially balance training; my new goal was to get to the course as healthy as possible. I would not try to develop new skills or strength. I just wanted to get there and be as much of me as I could over the next few days before the competition. I felt like I was only 50 percent of the fresh, trained, ninja Chris Warnky.

Daily, as I improved, I continued to check my hip, and sure enough, it just took several days for the bruising to appear. And boy did it appear! It was very large and dark, changing colors day by day as it progressed through the healing process. I finally felt validated about how much my hip was hurting. Based on where it was located I didn't share it with anyone but Carolyn. She helped me deal with the pain and had an appreciation for how bad the bruise was.

I continued to be careful during the remaining days in line. By the time of the competition I was much closer to normal, and I was so thankful. But this little injury had added to the challenges I faced during the walk-on-line experience.

Slack Line in the Park

A couple of times our gang went to a park and set up a slack line. Slack lines weren't in my current training routine other than a 10-foot-long version at Movement Lab Ohio. Even now I'm not consistent in crossing it successfully. I have attempted to cross it over 1,000 times. Jesse reminds me that I'm only 9,000 attempts away from being really good at it.

The longer 30-foot slack lines, where the ends are tied to tree trunks, and where the bounce is so much greater, are currently out of my league. If I really want to learn this skill, I need to spend a lot more time working with long slack lines.

It was helpful to get tips from walk-on-line members who are slack-line experts, including Steve, Danny, Noel, Julien, and Bryce. It was fun to watch them walk across the 20 or 30 feet, turn around, do a one-footed squat, and so many other moves while remaining on the line. They were impressive!

A Bag of Oranges

Ninja friend Shanon Paglieri tells me, "If you're starting to feel a cold coming on, eat a whole bag of oranges." I haven't liked oranges, not because of the taste but because they are messy to eat. Since I was living out of my car that made eating oranges even more of a challenge. At one point when I was trying everything I thought could help, I decided to try the "bag of oranges" approach. I found a grocery store in Grand Lakes and bought a full bag of oranges. I didn't have an orange cutter/peeler, so I bought a cheap fruit knife with a plastic safety sheath. I also bought some wet wipes, which I knew I would need if I tried to eat the oranges in or near my car.

I reached out to Shanon to get some tips about how best to peel and eat oranges, but her best advice was to use a bunch of paper towels. I did successfully eat two oranges in my car without staining the seats. I ate another two oranges at a picnic table. But I didn't get through the whole bag as she had proposed. I can only hope they helped.

I was trying so many remedies at the same time that it was hard to know what was or was not making a difference – I just needed help to get over that cold! The good news was that within five days I was over it. Thanks, Shanon, for your oranges recommendation.

Walk-On-Line Shirts from Scott

On my fifth day in line ninja Scott Reuter joined us. He was very engaging with our group. After our morning check-in he made a comment about getting shirts made and that he was hoping some of us would pitch in. He headed off to his car, and I hadn't really understood what he meant.

That evening we learned what he had been up to all day. He had a bunch of shirts printed with the *ANW* logo on the front and the words "Cleveland 2017 Walk-Ons." On the back he listed the names of the walk-ons who had joined the line to that point. He listed us in order of our place in line. He also slipped in the name of our senior casting producer at the end of the list.

They looked great and were a lot of fun. He had more than enough for each of us to get one. He asked that if possible we contribute to the cost of the shirts, which were very inexpensive. I purchased mine right away. It looked great and would help me commemorate the experience for the rest of my life. Thanks, Scott, for taking the initiative.

I wore this shirt on the city finals night and received a number of silver signatures on the shirt from the many ninjas and fans who were there celebrating my run on the qualifying course. It was so fun to open my coat, reveal my shirt, hand a silver Sharpie® to a ninja or fan, and have them sign my shirt while I stretched out my arms, firmed up my stomach, and held my breath. I have signatures all over the front and sides, and even some on the back. I cherish this shirt, and especially the silver signatures that pop on that beautiful black shirt. Again, thanks Scott.

Check-In with Michael Moore

Texas ninja and friend Michael Moore would call and check in with me on how things were going with my walk-on-line experience. I had met Michael a few years earlier in Las Vegas at an *ANW* finals competition. He's just a few months younger than I, and I featured him and his ninja story in *The Heart of a Ninja*.

He asked questions and shared a few of his walk-on-line stories and experiences. It's always good to get a call from Michael because he's so encouraging.

I shared with him some of the challenges I was facing with my cold and my hip bruise. He challenged me by telling me that I was not going to develop any cool new skills in the last few days before the competition. He said, "Don't push anything at this point. Don't get hurt. Just be healthy and ready to be the best you can be on Monday night with the hundreds of training hours you've already invested in the past three years."

It was great to have Michael calling and checking in with me through this experience.

The Coveted Producer Call

On May 2nd, Tuesday night, some ninjas in our line reported that they had received a call from an *ANW* producer who asked for information to use if they were to run the course and be aired on NBC. This was an exciting time for our group. These calls helped us feel like *ANW* had seen our names on our walk-on list, just as Julien had told us they had. They knew who we were. We weren't taking a gamble that was unknown to *ANW*.

We were very clear about our line order, so we were quite sensitive as to who would be or should be called next, but at least one of us was called out of order. That played with his head for a little while. He thought maybe he had been skipped. But a call came in to him as well, just a little later than he had expected. I don't know how this worked; it could have been multiple producers calling us and one reached a particular ninja earlier than the others.

At 6:22 p.m. I had just finished eating at a local sandwich shop and was getting back into my car when my phone rang. The call was from the 310 area code, which I wasn't familiar with. I paused for a moment. I don't often take calls when I don't know who they're from. And it was not the *ANW* 818 area code from California that's known by all ninjas who hope to get invited to compete on the show. But I went ahead and answered the phone.

The caller introduced himself by name and then stated he was an *ANW* producer. He asked if I was indeed in the walk-on line. He then asked if I was available to answer a few questions. I quickly assured him, "Yes, I would be happy to answer some questions."

He was friendly and conversational. He asked if there was anything new about me that he should know. I asked if he was looking for content that was new since my mid-December submission video and application. He said, "Yes, that's what I'm looking for."

Thinking on my feet, although I was actually sitting in my car with the door still open, I answered, "Yes. I think there are two or three things that may be of interest." I shared how I was now writing a book, *The Heart of a Ninja*, about my ninja warrior training experience. I told him I had been the Facebook Livestream announcer for the NNL Finals competition in California. I also shared that I was now conducting Ninja Lite classes at MLAB OH. He was interested in all three of these updates and asked for more detail about each of them. He wanted to know what caused me to be engaged with each, how they had gone or were going, and how I benefited from each of them.

My call with the producer lasted 15 minutes. I shared a good deal of content with him without running on too much. It was a fun and encouraging call, and validation that I was a member of the *ANW* walk-on line.

I was excited that a producer had really called and asked about me. My creative juices started to flow and best-case-scenario stories started to play in my mind. I could get to run the course! They could show my run on NBC! They could talk about my new ninja book, which would be a fantastic promotion or at least get the word out that the book was coming. I started

• 85 •

thinking about how my publishing timing would work with this possible NBC exposure, and whether I could get future opportunities to announce for other ninja competitions with other gyms and leagues. I could even have some fun time in the NBC booth, joining Matt and Akbar. And maybe this would open up opportunities to work with many other new ninjas in a ninja-lite way, helping them get on ninja obstacles and play and move. That could be a blast! My mind was going gangbusters with the possibilities. I was in overdrive with best-case scenarios. I had to be careful not to be too optimistic, but it was a blast to think about the possibilities, especially after being in the line for over a week with only a hope that it would lead to running the course.

It didn't take long to take a breath, step back, and say to myself, "Hey, this is great. A producer has your name. He called you and wanted to know a little more about you. Those are the facts. Don't get carried away." To ensure that I was grounded in my thinking I added, "You don't even know if you'll be on the official *ANW* walk-on line – it doesn't start till 10:00 a.m. Wednesday morning. Take this one step at a time, Mr. Chris. Slow down. There are still a lot of steps before you'll have a chance to run on the course."

I shared with our gang on our Messenger string, "I just got my producer call!" This was becoming more real all the time.

A Bonus

Being in downtown Cleveland, I continually tried to find the best way to use my time between check-ins. My health, the weather, and activities with the other ninjas were always key factors.

On Sunday the 30th of April, Scott and I decided to go to the early afternoon Cleveland Indians and Seattle Mariners baseball game. It was a beautiful day, and it was an early game so we would easily make it back for our 5:00 p.m. check-in. As it worked out, that was the one day the walk-ons agreed to skip the 5:00 p.m. check-in, so there was even less pressure to stick to a schedule. It was a great game. The Indians destroyed the Mariners, winning 12 to 4, and were in the lead for most of the game.

We saw several home runs with fireworks celebrations for each of them. Our seats were in the top row of the stadium, almost directly behind home plate. It was very windy, but that made our shaded seats even more comfortable. We watched this fun competition for over three hours. Scott had played baseball in high school and college, and it was fun to talk some baseball with him, which I hadn't done for years. It was a special bonus to my Cleveland time.

After all of that waiting, the official *ANW* walk-on line was formed, which you will learn about in the next chapter.

Chapter 8

The Official *ANW* Line Forms

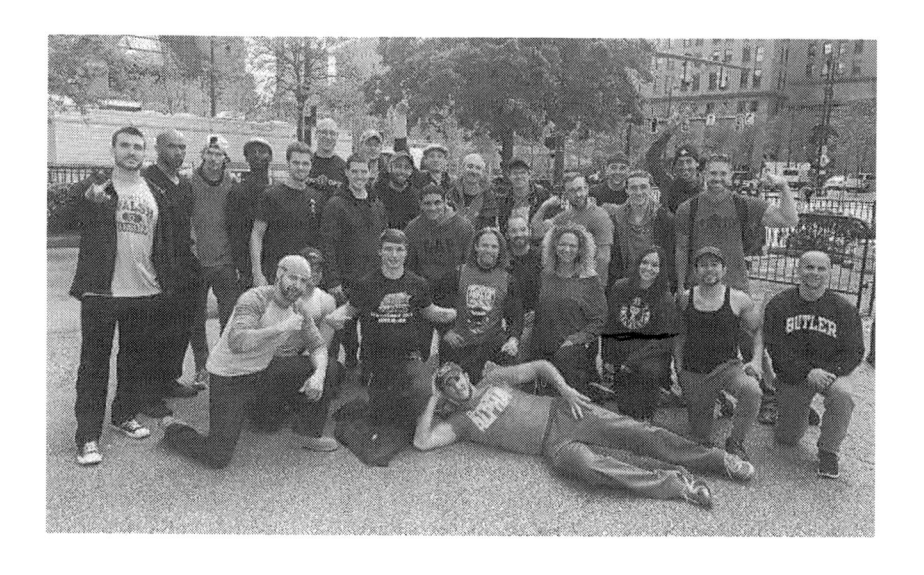

On my ninth day in line we received word that *ANW* had posted information about the start of the official Cleveland walk-on line. All that we had sacrificed for so far was unofficial activity. I eventually found that the information stated the following:

- The line would start at 10:00 a.m. and be firmed up by noon.
- Not to be on *ANW* designated property in advance of 10:00.
- Not to loiter in a public area.

We wanted the transition to the official line to go as smoothly as possible. Now that the whole world knew where and when to show up (it was posted on the internet), we tried to figure out how best to approach the official start time. We didn't want other ninjas to show up and form another line early the next morning, so we had to determine how to solidify our position and at the same time not loiter and not be on *ANW* property.

We decided to be at the designated area five hours early, at 5:00 a.m. We hoped that as other ninjas showed up we could explain that we already had an established line that they could join, but we didn't know – or at least I didn't know – how it would actually work.

Again, my mind started creating all kinds of scenarios, this time with all the negative things that could happen. I asked myself, "Are there going to be other ninjas showing up and creating a line at midnight or earlier? Are there going to be thirty people in line when we show up at five o'clock? Are there going to be arguments between like-minded competitive ninjas who are all trying to get in line? Is there going to be another line of fifty ninjas who met up somewhere else in the area and come walking up to the official spot at ten o'clock? After all the time we have already invested in this process, what will happen?"

Some in our line felt it would be fine to show up at 8:00, two hours early. Others, like me, weren't sure that even 5:00 was early enough. Ninjas who have trained for so long and so hard really want to have the opportunity to run the course; they might get there very early. We finally agreed on meeting at 5:00.

There were mixed feelings about where we should park, and discussion about if and when we could get out of our cars prior to 10:00. No one wanted to put any of our invested time at risk. It was so hard to know what we could and should do. For me, a planner type of guy, it was an extremely frustrating and confusing few hours.

To the Site

I woke very early and arrived at the designated spot at 4:45 a.m., a little early. It was a public parking lot. It was still dark and would be for a couple more hours. I pulled up to the booth at the entrance and told the attendant I was with the *ANW* walk-on line. He said okay, did not charge me for parking, and directed me to an area of the parking lot where there were orange cones. I drove there, pulled into a tight spot in an area behind the cones, and sat there waiting for the rest of our gang to show up. I had not seen the official walk-on-line communication that warned to stay out of the designated *ANW* area.

After about 15 minutes I saw Messenger comments about others also being there, but I couldn't see anyone. I got out of my car and wandered in the dark looking for where they were. I saw a few cars on the other side of the cones in the public parking lot, and squinting in the dark I tried to see if they belonged to members of our line. I hadn't seen them earlier, and I thought they must have come after I had. I made my way over to one of the cars and sure enough it belonged to one of our members. Following a little small-talk, I asked them about where they were parked and told them where I was parked. One of their concerns was about not being on the *ANW* designated site. They strongly encouraged me to move my car to where they were. Squinting all the way in the darkness, I headed over to my car. I backed up, pulled around to the other side of a white tent, and found an opening in the cones, so I pulled through. I made my way slowly through the nearly empty, dark parking lot and backed in next to the others.

When I turned off my engine I could see that the parking lot attendant was heading my way. He asked me to roll down my window and said, "Hey, you know you owe me ten dollars, right?" In frustration I said, "I don't know what I'm supposed to be doing." He followed up with, "You owe me ten dollars!" Then he quickly headed back to his booth by the entrance.

I was still trying to figure out what the *ANW* guidelines meant. Where were we supposed to be and by when? Were we supposed to pay to be in this parking lot or not? I finally decided that if I was going to be on this side of the cones, I should probably pay. He must have thought I was a member of the *ANW* staff when he originally let me into the lot, and was not familiar with the walk-on-line concept.

Later I learned that each of the other ninjas had paid $10 to park there. I reasoned to myself, "Maybe paying the ten dollars is my proof that I'm on 'public property' as a patron and not in violation on '*ANW* property.'" If that was the case, when I got out of my car I would not technically be loitering, I would simply be standing in front of my car having paid to park. But I couldn't be confident about any option or decision I was making. It seemed to entail risk on one front or another.

I got out of my car, walked 80 feet over to the booth, offered the attendant a $10 bill, and told him I was sorry and that I really didn't know what was going on or what I was supposed to be doing. I asked him his name and he told me "Ernie." I asked what he knew about *ANW* and he said, "Very little." I shared with him a little about the walk-on-line experience and we chatted for about five minutes until it was time for him to check in the next car coming into the lot. Ernie seemed like a great guy who was trying to do his job well. He was charged to make money on every car he could get into that 300-car lot, and as I learned later, he did a great job of squeezing cars in everywhere he could. He's an expert at what he does and he's firm and respectful with each of his patrons.

The Need for Food and a Public Bathroom... Again

A little before 7:00 a.m. on that early Wednesday morning, a small group of us headed out to find food and a bathroom. We crossed Public Square and headed down Euclid, looking for somewhere that was open and could provide some warm food.

It was still very cool. We walked several blocks hoping for a diner where we could sit for a few minutes in the warmth, eat some hot food, and use the bathroom, but such a place did not turn up.

We finally found a little shop that had hot food. I ordered a large, very hot egg gyro. It tasted great! It felt so good and warm inside. I also got an orange juice to help with both my dry mouth and my cold/semi-sore-throat. The shop had a couple of small tables but only four chairs, so we took turns sitting and eating our breakfasts before we headed back. There was no restroom, which was becoming a much bigger priority for a few of us, especially me.

On the way back we stopped at the JACK Cleveland Casino, went through the "carding" process with the guard, and went quickly and directly to the men's restroom. The only gambling we were doing was to see if we could get to the bathroom in time. I was proud of the fact that none of us ran. After finishing this critical business we walked right past that same guard and back outside and back to our cars, and Scott joined me in my car.

At one point I left my car to talk to a few of the ninjas while Scott stayed behind. A little later, when he got out of the car and closed the door, somehow he set off the car alarm. I don't know why it went on or how it eventually got turned off, but it was a big surprise to Scott.

Additional Ninjas Show Up

Around 7:00 a.m. a few people began to stroll into the parking lot. Firmly and confidently, Julien would get out of his car and approach each one to find out if they were in the area to join the ninja walk-on line. If so, he then shared that a walk-on line had formed and that they could be added to "the book" — our unofficial yet as official as we could make it book — to get the next available number. This seemed to work well. Over the next three hours our list grew slowly and peaceably from 19 to 27. I was so relieved to see this work so well. My tension started to lessen.

While we were waiting I invited Scott and Bryce to join me and wait in my car. They had both parked across the street in another lot to ensure they were not on the official *ANW* walk-on-line property. They were even a little paranoid about sitting in my car in that lot. And for all I knew their paranoia might be justified. But Julien, our multiyear walk-on-line leader, was also parked in this lot, so I hoped we were okay. The three of us visited for over an hour while we closely watched and evaluated the activity taking place in the parking lot with Julien and the other ninjas parked there.

By 9:30, 30 minutes prior to the start of the official *ANW* walk-on line, most of us had stepped out of our cars and were standing in front of them. We had our official book. We now had 27 walk-on names in show-up order in the book. No one seemed to be concerned about standing in a particular order. We were huddled in small clusters anticipating what would be next and introducing ourselves to those who were new to the line.

A little after 10:00 the senior casting producer came walking across the street, heading toward us. This was the first time we had seen him during this multiday process. I recognized him from so many other ninja events. He was always directing ninja traffic on the sidelines. He also recognized me, not only from my submission video but also from the many hours I spent on the sidelines of ninja events.

Senior-Casting-Producer Time

Our senior casting producer approached Julien and received hugs from several ninjas who knew him quite well. He greeted us, asked Julien for the book with the vital list of names, now numbering 29 ninjas, and directed us to the white tent that I had driven around five hours earlier.

Once we were inside he welcomed us again and distributed blank profile sheets for each of us to complete. Those of us who had pens quickly completed our form and lent our pen to someone who didn't have one. The tent was a holding area that would later be set up with tables and chairs. At this point there were just a bunch of folded and stacked six-foot-long tables and some chair stands holding 100 or so folding chairs. There weren't many flat surfaces available to write on so we all scrambled for either someone else's back or one of the racks of stacked tables, writing on the flat surfaces in between the folded legs.

Julien had done a great job managing our list but he hadn't asked for our email addresses, which were also needed, so we began the process of writing all of those on a sheet of paper.

One of the ninjas, being helpful and hoping to get a few extra brownie points, offered to enter the names, phone numbers, and email addresses into the senior casting producer's computer. We continued standing and waiting for this process to be completed.

The senior casting producer exchanged fun ninja stories with us and answered questions during this time, which lasted about 40 minutes. Then he collected our completed forms, gave us instructions, and answered questions like "How many family and friends do we get to bring to the site for our run?" and "Where do we need to be next?" He then led us outside where he took a quick head-shot photo of each of us in the order we were in the book. This went smoothly and quickly until number eight, who was away at the bathroom. Throughout those weeks together our number order was a critical and sensitive topic. No one wanted to do anything to jeopardize their place in line. We each had worked way too hard to give up even one spot. One spot, as I already shared, could make a difference in whether or not a ninja would get to run on the course. We were all thankful that he simply skipped her and came back to her at the end, and it didn't have a negative impact on her place in line.

Then he asked us to pose for a full group photo and video. We had fun displaying energy and enthusiasm in the video and in a couple of the photos.

After the photos he dismissed us with the direction to come back on Sunday for some video footage of our walk-on line. He said he would email details once they were available. With that we were done.

We Are Official!

The first big walk-on-line hurdle was having our number order documented and confirmed. Done! It was amazing to me how much relief I felt to have made this hurdle after the initial memorable 10-day investment. I discovered immediately that I was hungry and extremely exhausted. The ambiguity had really taxed me mentally and emotionally.

Before we disbursed, many of our original walk-ons headed over to another area and took a fun video and some photos together. I was talking to one of the ninjas who had arrived that morning and didn't hear about that photo session till after the fact, so unfortunately I was not included in those shots.

This was already quite a long day. I was headed home, but I stopped for a celebration meal at Five Guys Burgers and Fries. I was starved and wanted to celebrate this big milestone with a large portion of great-tasting French fries, which are probably my number-one celebration food — maybe even ahead of ice cream.

Then I headed out of town toward home. Less than an hour into my two-hour drive I pulled into a rest area, rolled down my windows, reclined in my seat, and fell asleep for nearly an hour because I was so exhausted from those 10 days. I really needed that nap! When I woke I was able to drive the rest of the way home. It was so good to be home and to see Carolyn again.

To this point the walk-on-line experience had been all about waiting. On Sunday morning things really started to happen. In the next chapter you will see how I juggled our plans and the new challenges that surfaced.

Chapter 9

A Busy Sunday Morning

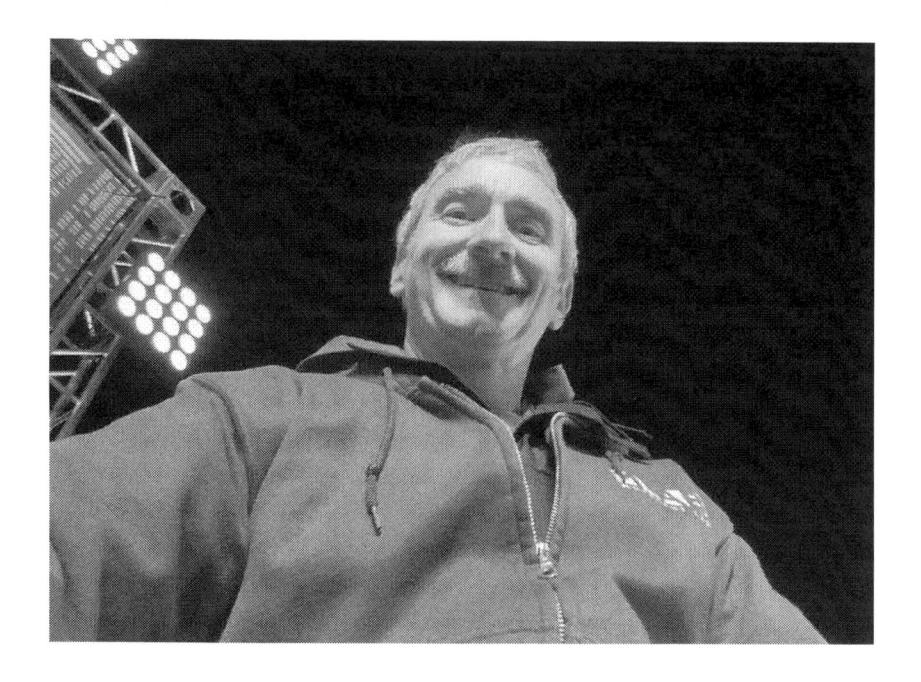

We didn't need to report back to Cleveland until Sunday at noon, which was a nice surprise; I had not anticipated a break at home, which provided me with three nights to recover in my own bed.

During the MLAB OH Friday noon open gym I worked out with a number of ninjas, several of whom were Cleveland *ANW* invitees. I heard my phone ring, went to check it, and noticed it was an unfamiliar number. I said the area code out loud and the ninjas quickly blurted out, "Pick it up! Pick it up! It's *ANW*!"

I answered the phone, and sure enough the call was from someone at *ANW* asking if I could be at an interview in downtown Cleveland on Sunday morning at 7:30. That was definitely going to be "bright and early," before breakfast or church. A couple of days earlier Michelle had mentioned that a producer had called to asked if I would be available for an interview on Sunday. They wanted to ask me about Michelle and some other ninja friends, especially Shanon Paglieri. Carolyn and I had planned to be in Cleveland on Saturday (the next day) to visit Tim and his family and celebrate Carolyn's birthday, so this interview would have to fit on top of our already planned wild-and-crazy ninja and family activities. (Carolyn, I hope you feel you were celebrated, loved, and appreciated even though we had so much other activity going on on your birthday!)

I told the woman calling from *ANW*, "Yes, I can be available." She was relieved and excited that I could make that time slot. She was probably also coordinating with many other ninjas to fill interview slots.

I understood that this was an interview about Michelle, Shanon, and others, not about me. It would be fun, and I was looking forward to talking about these great ninjas who are family or good friends who feel like family.

Carolyn and I drove to Tim's on Saturday morning and had a nice visit with him and his family. We also had a nice dinner out that evening as a birthday celebration for Carolyn, and spent the night at Tim's home.

To My Sunday Morning Interview

I woke up very early Sunday morning so I could start my trek downtown by 6:40 a.m. I wanted to make sure I was there by at least 7:20. It was about a 30-minute drive and I had to find the parking lot and walk to the hotel where the interviews were taking place.

I like to make sure I get to commitments early. I want to be sure I'll be there on time even if I experience a road being closed, an accident, road construction, getting lost, or whatever. My reputation is to be on time or early, and usually early.

When I arrived at the parking lot on that bright and sunny Sunday morning I noticed and then waved to a guy a couple of parking spots away. He looked familiar. We recognized each other as being ninjas, so we shared our names and shook hands. His name was Patrick Lavanty. After sharing a good-luck wish with him, I headed toward the hotel. On my way I came across another ninja friend, Logan Broadbent, "The Boomerang" ninja, who was also arriving for an early-morning interview. He was collecting his gear from his car, so after a quick "Hi" and hug, I was again headed toward the hotel. He would be there soon.

To the *American Ninja Warrior* Room

As I stepped into the ornate Renaissance Hotel, I headed to the concierge to ask for directions to the *American Ninja Warrior* room. He directed me down the hall and told me which turns to make. I don't know if it was my excitement or lack of sleep over the past few weeks, but I walked past the room. I did come across another vital room – I stopped at the men's restroom to use the facility and check my hair. I wanted to make sure everything was relatively in place for my upcoming interview.

When I came out of the men's room I saw a couple of familiar women ninjas in the hall. They knew where we were supposed to go, so I followed them back down the hall and into a large ballroom. A production staffer approached us with her clipboard with names and times. She asked each of us our name, checked it off, and sent us to a designated place.

There were chairs set up along the perimeter of the two long sides of the room. There were plenty of chairs, but the center of the room was empty. I headed to a chair on the side closest to the door and set down my backpack. I started to engage with the other ninjas who were already there. Those I already knew got a quick hug and a "Great to see you." Those I did not recognize, or did not yet know, got a quick smile and either a wave or a handshake as my ninja community continued to grow by the minute.

My Group Is Called

After a few minutes of interaction, six of us were called and another assistant led us back to the hallway and toward the elevators. We were taken to the sixth floor and instructed to take a seat in one of the six folding chairs that were set up in a small lobby just across from the elevator. It was a standard hotel-room floor and it looked like we were going to be interviewed in hotel rooms specifically set up for the interviews.

There must have been several interview rooms and producers. One at a time a producer would appear, introduce themselves, and escort one of us to an interview room. We learned more about each other as ninjas as we waited there in the lobby for our interviews.

Peggy Hale, one of the MLAB OH ninjas I train with, was in our interview group. Michael Nowoslawski, our number-one walk-on-line ninja who received the Golden Ticket to compete was also in our group. McKinley Peirce, whom I met at the NNL finals in California, was also in our group. McKinley had had a great NNL year, coming in third among the women in the finals.

I took my normal self-assigned role of introducing those I already knew to each other and to those I was meeting for the first time. It's so fun to learn the background and story of each ninja. It only took a few minutes for each of us to open up and share a little of our story.

My Interview

Eventually a producer called my name and led me off to my interview room. I was the third one called from our group. As we walked down the hall we had a short conversation about him, me, and the interview process that was to take place around the corner. We walked past a guy sitting just outside the door who was wearing a headset and adjusting some equipment. I later learned that he was the audio engineer who would ensure the recording was just right and that no loud sounds were made in the hallway that would interfere with a good quality interview.

My interview was scheduled for 7:30, but it didn't start until 45 minutes later – and these were the early interviews; I can't imagine what the timing must have been like for the interviews scheduled for later in the day. Carolyn and I had planned on joining Tim and his family at Parkside Church in Chagrin Falls for the 9:30 service, and I was starting to wonder if I was going to make it. Flexibility had been so important over the first 14 days of my walk-on-line experience, and this was going to be another instance in which I would have to just see what happened.

I took off my coat, and as we began to set up for the interview I asked if the shirt I was wearing was okay. The instructions provided for the interview were very specific about what were and were not appropriate colors and what I should and should not wear; for example, the instructions said "no green." To be safe I had brought several shirt options. I was wearing the shirt I would run in on Monday night. It was my black "This Is What a Really Cool 60 Year Old Looks Like" shirt. The instructions specifically said "don't wear black," but I wanted to go in wearing my special shirt. I began to pull out my other shirts, which included a plain red T-shirt and several of the shirts I planned to wear Monday night to support my ninja friends during their runs on the course. I was expecting to be asked about a few of these ninjas in the interview. My shirt stack included my "Shantastic," "Pocket Ninja," and "Ickfisch" shirts, which each represented a fellow ninja and friend who had been invited to run the course. But the producer said my special black shirt would be just fine. That made me very happy, and it was a great way to start the interview.

The Setup

I was directed to a rectangular wooden box sitting upright in the center of the room. It stood about two-and-a-half feet tall with a one-foot by one-foot base. This was where I was to sit. It was positioned perfectly for the camera. This was a very well planned and efficient interview process. They would probably record 15 or more interviews that day in just that one room.

Next to me was another wooden box. This one was lying down horizontally, with an "X" taped across the top. The X indicated where the cold bottle of water was to be placed for my interview. They offered the bottle of water to me so that I would have a nice wet throat when I started speaking. I took the bottle, unscrewed the lid, took a nice long swig, screwed the cap back on, and placed the bottle right in the center of the X on the box. What precision by this aspiring ninja interviewee!

The producer asked me to focus directly on him and not to pay any attention to the equipment or other people in the dark room. The equipment included a gigantic white light, a white reflector screen directly in front of my face, and a huge microphone placed close to the top of my head, just out of camera view. In the dark background, beyond the producer, I could see the camera that would record my comments.

"Just focus on me. Talk to me," he said. I've been on camera a lot, both through my radio-and-TV-broadcasting college education and through my years as a corporate video producer and on-camera talent. I zeroed in on his face and we were ready to go.

After a couple of my comments the camera guy said, "We need to move the white reflector; it's in the shot." What they did not know was that this interviewee is a guy who can be quite animated, with many facial and body expressions, including shoulder shrugs, straightening, slouching, and leaning to the left and the right and forward and backward. I move and express myself. When I made a key point I would sit up straighter, extend my eyebrows, and move my head higher than the camera view, so the cameraman had to pan upward, revealing the bottom of the reflector in his shot. After a few adjustments to move the reflector up just a little, we were set to go.

The Interview

After stating my name and age, we were on to the producer's key questions. (I had hoped you would be able to hear some of my fun responses on NBC during the Cleveland *ANW* city qualifier episode, but none of them were used.) I had been instructed to speak in complete sentences, not just respond to the questions. In other words, if the question was "How impressed are you with Michelle's accomplishments?" they didn't want me to respond, "I'm very impressed," but rather, "I'm very impressed with Michelle's accomplishments." I was able to answer each of his questions in relatively short, complete, stand-alone statements, and there were very few retakes.

The questions he asked were as they had stated. I talked about Michelle being my daughter and the inspiration she has been to me and so many other ninjas, especially women and kids. I was asked about how excited I was to have *ANW* in Cleveland. I was also asked how Michelle felt about competing in Cleveland. Michelle and I had never talked about that, but the camera was rolling, so I told them what she might have said to me if we had talked about it. I shared that she was excited to have *ANW* come to her own backyard, Cleveland, Ohio – her home state – where many family and friends could cheer her on and celebrate with her.

He asked me about my number-one training partner (NOTP), Shanon Paglieri. We talked about her growth, her skill, and her physical challenges and limitations, though I didn't know much about her physical limitations at that time. And he asked how well I thought Shanon would do on the course. I enjoyed talking about how strong she had become due to her dedication and work ethic. She worked so hard over an extended period, and it paid off in her performances. It's so much fun to watch her compete and enjoy the courses!

Shanon and I were much closer in skill level when we started to train, which was three years before that. I have grown so much during my first three to four years, but Shanon has moved to a whole new level, way beyond me on so many obstacles. At times I get jokingly frustrated with her performances, especially on upper-body and balance obstacles, because she has become so strong. It amazes me and frustrates me because I'm not yet where she is, but I'm so, so happy for her.

As expected, the focus was on Michelle, Shanon, and the city of Cleveland. He did ask a few questions about my being Michelle's dad. The whole interview was completed within 10 minutes.

Then the producer stood up, walked around the light and reflector, gave me a nice firm handshake, and said, "Great job. I wish you well in your potential course run."

I picked up my bottle of water and jested, "I'm guessing you'll use a new bottle for your next interviewee." With a grin the producer responded, "For sure." I picked up my stuff and was led out the door, past the audio man, and down the hall again to the lobby where a few of the remaining ninjas were still waiting. My interview was done. Next on the agenda was our video shoot.

Missed Church Again

I had planned to join my family at church in Chagrin Falls, grab lunch with Carolyn, and drop her off at the hotel we would be staying at Sunday night before getting to the *ANW* video shoot at noon, but I ended up missing almost all of the church service, which was disappointing. Carolyn and I said a quick good-bye to Tim's family and went to lunch at Chipotle, then I dropped her off at the hotel and got to the video shoot with just 10 minutes to spare.

Whew! It's time to take a breath, then we're on to the official walk-ons video shoot in the next chapter.

Chapter 10

The Walk-Ons Video Shoot

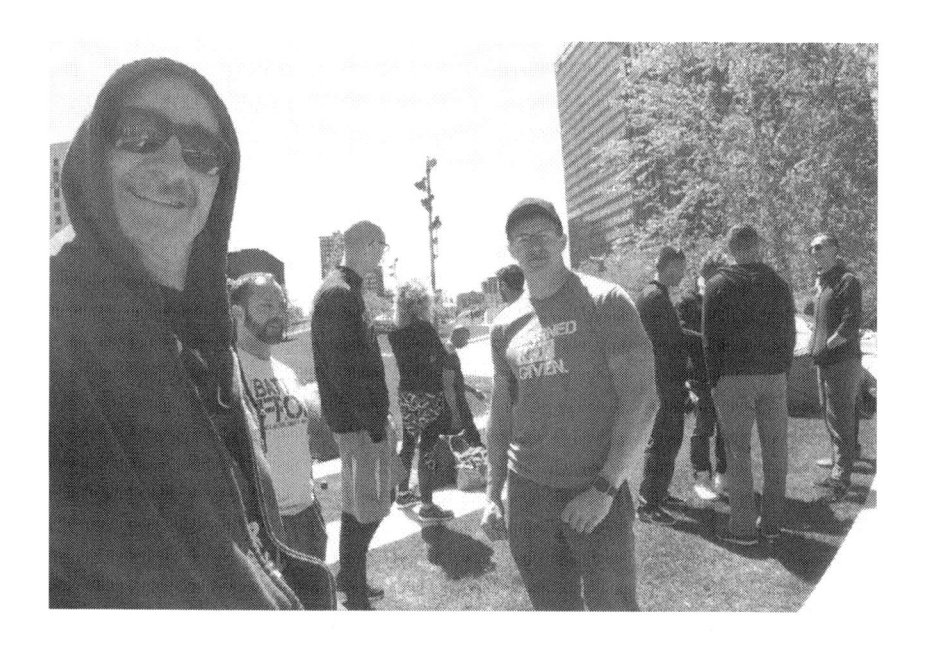

I took my CamelBak® backpack and some food to munch on and joined the others at the designated parking area for the video shoot. Our senior casting producer had told us he didn't know how long the shoot would take, but to be prepared for several hours and he would dismiss us as soon as he could.

He arrived at the parking lot, led us over to the course, and created an opening in the portable fence rails so we could walk into the site. We were on the actual *ANW* course site for the very first time. This was really happening! It felt good to be "inside."

He started to search for an area that was just close enough to the course so that it would be in the background. We walked to the top of a small landscaped hill with several concrete terraces facing Public Square.

It was a beautiful day. The sun was shining brightly and there were a few bright, white clouds in the sky, enough to give it real character. I was wearing my old "BattleFrog" brimmed hat to keep from getting too much sun on my face and neck. I also loaded up with high-SPF suntan lotion because I had some skin cancer removed from the back of my neck a few years ago and have been protective of my skin since then.

Another producer came with a camera to document ninjas in various activities across the field. A slack line was set up between two medium-sized trees. Some balance obstacles were also set up. A football was being thrown back and forth across the field. Ninja Jesse Wildman even played his guitar. Other ninjas stood around in small groups shooting the breeze about the process and what was yet to come.

During this time testing was occurring on the *ANW* course. It was very hard not to look, stare, and study what was happening. Technically we weren't supposed to be looking, but it was very hard not to see how the testers were doing. The goal was to look but not look like we were looking. We could see some of the invited ninjas watching the testers from outside the fence, so we didn't feel too bad about the view we were getting. Most of us studied the obstacles during the next two or three hours. Scott Reuter had brought his grill, some charcoal, hot dogs, condiments, and plates. It was a fun twist that Scott brought to our group.

The producer would call the name of a ninja he wanted to interview or film in an action shot or both. He also recorded the hot dogs cooking on the grill and many other activities. I don't believe I was recorded in any of the activity shots that were taken. I stayed on one of the top terraces talking with a few other ninjas. I had already been in an interview and wasn't seeking more camera exposure like many of the others. It's fun to be on TV and I understand the desire to get the exposure, but for whatever reason — maybe I was just too worn out — I didn't try to get in the videos at that time.

At one point the producer had us all line up and cheer "Cleveland rocks!" as he panned through the entire line of Cleveland walk-on ninjas. He recognized me and introduced himself as the guy who had called that Tuesday night. It was great to put a name and a face with his voice.

Near the end of the shoot that Sunday afternoon the focus was on getting a few final individual interviews. They were being conducted close to the course. Specific questions were being asked relative to either being in the walk-on line or the ninja's personal story.

Then I heard my name called. I jumped up and trotted down to the interview spot with the producer. I was surprised to be called since I had already been interviewed that morning. I was asked about my walk-on-line experience, being Michelle's dad, and being ready to run the course. It was simple, short, and sweet, and partially redundant of what I had shared with the other producer in the morning interview.

After the final interview was recorded, the senior casting producer called us together and told us we were free to go. He distributed parking vouchers, which we appreciated. His next message was, "See you Monday night at 5:00 p.m. sharp. Meet me at the corner of the fence, at the opposite side of the course from the Friends and Family check-in area."

We said our good-byes until Monday night, about 24 hours from then, and headed back to our cars. I took it easy and didn't rush. It was a very nice day and I was enjoying being there, outside, in that beautiful weather. After most of the ninjas had left, Jesse Wildman, Scott Walberry, me, and a few others were still wrapping up when we noticed a few of our MLAB OH testers walking along the outside of the fence north of the square. We trotted down to the fence to say hi and hear what they were planning to do next. Christy Baldwin had scraped her leg climbing on a statue. It was bleeding and hurting so she was ready to get some medical attention. We said good-bye for now, headed back up the hill, packed our things, left the fenced area, and walked across the first parking lot, across the street, and into the next lot to our cars.

We were down to the last 30 hours before the *ANW* Cleveland city qualifier would start. Time was flying now.

Chapter 11

Down to 30 Hours

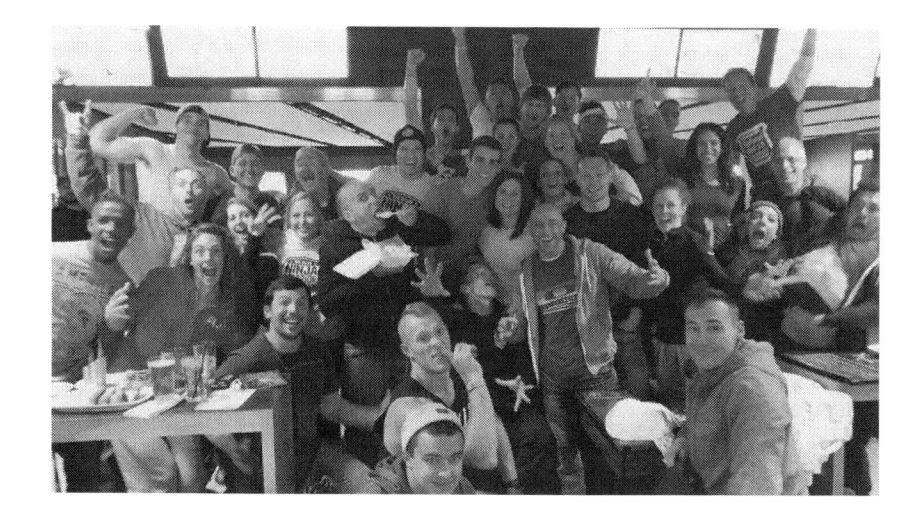

Throughout this experience I ran into ninjas everywhere. As we walked to our cars we spotted three more ninjas sitting in the back of a pickup truck waiting for the next round of testing. They were testing because they were either too young to compete, hadn't been invited to compete and did not want to get in the walk-on line, were just curious and wanted to get on the course, or had already run in another city and had not qualified for the Las Vegas finals. If you don't qualify you're eligible to test courses in other cities.

Most ninjas love to test anytime they are ineligible to run a course. There were a lot of strong ninja testers in Cleveland, the fifth city of the *ANW* season. Once you test a course you are no longer eligible to compete that season. There were several MLAB OH ninjas who had come to test in Cleveland, and it was great to see them there. Many of them did get on the course, but it was sad that some didn't.

I headed back to our hotel, and after a little catch-up time with Carolyn and a little rest we headed back to the course to see who was there, but most of the ninjas I knew had left the course by that time.

Late Dinner

Several of our MLAB OH ninjas had talked earlier about getting together for dinner. We found that Sunday night was not a good time to find restaurants open in Cleveland. Most catered to the work-week crowd. But we found a Winking Lizard several blocks away, and some of us headed there for a late dinner hoping to get there before they stopped serving. We made it there just in time before they stopped taking orders at 9:00.

We discovered that there's another Winking Lizard within walking distance from Public Square; when several ninjas seemed to be missing in action we texted them to find out where they were. They were also wondering where we were. They were at the other Winking Lizard, but there were 15 of us, which was plenty for our server, so we stayed put.

After dinner Carolyn and I walked back toward the course to see who was there, take another peek at the obstacles, and see if any additional testing was happening. Do you get the sense that we wanted to be by the course and around other ninjas? We sure did.

The next two nights we would be up all night so we didn't want to go to bed very early. Even though we ate a very late dinner and we also visited the course for a while, we still wanted to stay up. This was in sharp contrast to my normal bedtime of 9:00 or 10:00 p.m. (and often on the early side of that range!).

Sunday Night Bowling

Along with a host of other ninjas we had been invited by Kim Wenches, Jamie Rahn's fiancée at that time, to go bowling that night at 11:00 p.m. The bowling alley wasn't far from Public Square and was on the way to our hotel, so Carolyn and I decided to swing by and say hi. On our way Michelle and ninja Mike Bernardo caught up with us. There were already 15 ninjas bowling when we arrived. It looked like their goal was to have a lot of fun together, and they were doing just that. The screens mounted on the ceiling reflected low bowling scores. These guys and gals are great athletes, and kings and queens on their own turf, but not so much on the bowling lanes, at least not that night.

We enjoyed visiting for about an hour before we headed back to our hotel. By the time we left, over 25 ninjas had assembled. As often, we took a group picture to commemorate the experience.

Less Than 24 Hours to Go

In less than 24 hours some of us would have already run the qualifying course trying to advance to the finals. Some would have succeeded, some would have come up short, and some would still be waiting for other ninjas to run to find out if their distance and time was good enough to advance to the finals. Others would be sitting on the sidelines studying the performances of those who were running, waiting in anticipation for their shot to run a little later in the evening or early in the morning.

As we walked backed to the hotel my mind drifted to the fact that although Monday night would be night 34 for Carolyn and I to be at an *ANW* course, this one would be quite different for me. Just having the potential to run – whether I would run or not – would radically change my personal experience for the next day and night and for my future.

Just Enjoy It, Chris

I slept well that night. I was looking forward to this opportunity, whatever it was going to be. I was so excited for my friends who were going to be running the next night. This was going to be such a fun experience. "Just enjoy it, Chris — just enjoy it," I said to myself.

The big day was finally here. After all the preparation and waiting, what happened?

Chapter 12

I Have Learned So Much!

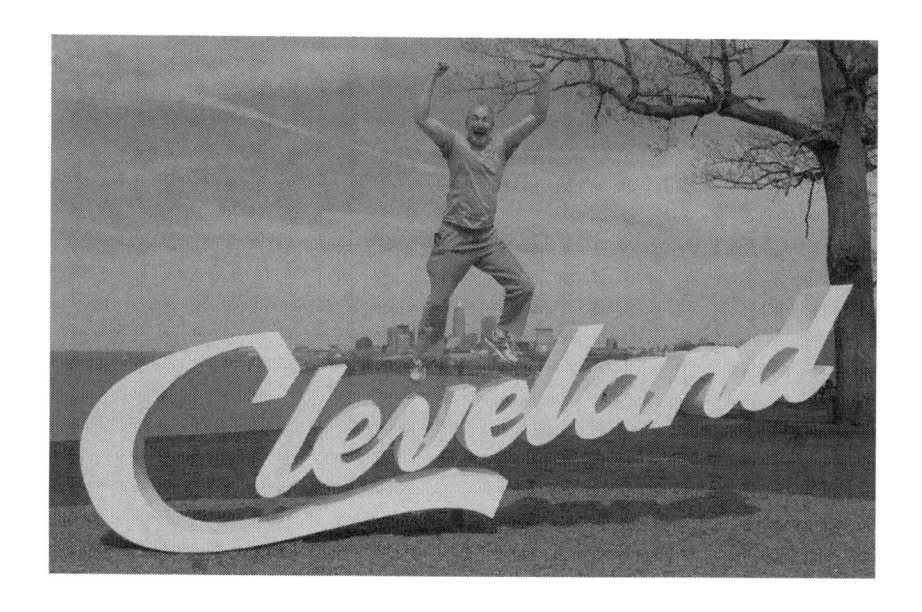

After a good night's sleep we did our best to manage the day knowing it was going to be a big night and a long, long one. We took it easy, fitting in more rest time, relaxing in the hot tub, filling out and signing the *ANW* legal forms, and finally packing and taking a short nap before we headed to the course.

I was sure to show up on time at our walk-on check-in location and went through all the steps of the ninja competition-night process, all the way to the point that it was time for me to run the course. There were multiple rounds of get-in-line-and-wait until we were finally taken to the holding tent where we joined the invited ninjas who were also waiting. We went through the course walk-through and then we waited to see if and when walk-ons would be called to run.

To my big surprise and relief, I did get to run the actual Cleveland *ANW* course on that cold night! It was quite an experience. There were several surprises along the way, but it did happen, and the whole night was a blast! It included so many fun twists.

I was also fortunate to be one of the few ninjas shown on NBC that night. Less than 30 percent of the ninjas who ran the course were shown on the episode. The anticipation of being shown on NBC is an experience in and of itself. The day of the filming, and being at our Cleveland episode-watch party, was so emotional; I hadn't known what to expect.

In my next book, *What Just Happened?: The Run: An* American Ninja Warrior *Cleveland Course-Run Experience* (targeted to be available on Amazon.com in 2019), I share my full experience from waking up the day of my course run through the airing of the NBC Cleveland city qualifier episode. There are so many interesting stories and surprises that happened, and they provided me with many high and low emotional experiences. I'm sure this was the same for many ninjas that night and throughout the

American Ninja Warrior years. I'm excited to share each of these experiences in full detail so you can feel what it's like to run an *ANW* course.

Lessons Learned

I love this statement from author John C. Maxwell: "Experience is not the greatest teacher, but rather evaluated experience." Here are a few of my key thoughts from evaluating this walk-on-line experience, and some of the lessons I learned:

- You can learn from every experience.
- The more experiences you have the more lessons you can potentially learn.
- Think before you act.
- Evaluate all your options — or at least as many as possible.
- Consider your big-picture goals and dreams and ensure that a potential experience can help you move toward them.
- Focus on what you can control, not on what is out of your control.
- Ensure that you can be content with both a best-case and a worst-case result.
- Open a door and you will experience more — sometimes more than you ever dreamed.
- Be patient and flexible. These traits are so important in life.

- Be committed to your goal and see it through to the best of your ability until you meet it.
- Be patient when time drags on. It's worth the wait.
- Most other people would like the best for you.
- The ninja community is a supportive, fun, and diverse group of people of many different ages from many different walks of life, providing great opportunities to learn from them.
- Take some calculated risks that are not guaranteed. It can help you stretch and grow. You miss so much when you do only what you feel is safe. Step outside your comfort zone.

Go After Your Dreams

The ninja warrior experience is just one of my goals or dreams. I have many. What dream or dreams are you currently chasing? I hope you have at least one dream, if not many, driving you forward. It's fun and rewarding to pursue and see progress in our lives, especially in areas that are most important to us.

Count the Cost and Make a Decision

I boldly and confidently drove to Cleveland that Sunday afternoon because I had taken the time to evaluate the cost of the experience and the potential return on my investment. After considering the best-case and worst-case scenarios I was ready to make a decision and take the appropriate actions. I didn't look back. I had done my homework and it paid off.

And I did experience many of these worst-case and best-case scenarios. In the end, both my experiences and the final results were more often best-case scenarios, and for this I am very thankful.

Focus on What You Control, and Be Content

Give your goals all your effort and then be content with the results. It's so important to be content in all situations — to be flexible and willing to change course and go with the flow. There is so much in your life that you don't control. Knowing this and being content in all situations is a powerful approach that changes your whole life experience. It can make challenges much more tolerable and potentially even enjoyable. Be content.

Living the Experience

I'm intrigued by the Mark Twain statement: "I've suffered a great many catastrophes in my life. Most of them never happened." When you create a picture in your mind it leads you to an emotional response and physical actions that are just like living the experience, even if it never happens.

I've been working to eliminate these fear-based images from my mind and focus on the facts in front of me. It really pays off when I do this. I get to experience reality, not the scary and fear-based possibilities that can shut me down and so limit my life.

These are a few of the key lessons I have learned. It was helpful to reflect on and be reminded of them as I wrote *What Just Happened?: The Line*, and I hope you were able to find examples of them throughout the book.

Pinch Me

This was an unbelievable experience! When I slow down and think about it I can still hardly believe I went through the 16-day walk-on-line experience. It all started just a little before that moment when I asked Carolyn, "What if I were to join the walk-on line?"

This experience was not cheap when I consider the hours, the dollars, the training, and the aggravation I went through up through my run and all that followed. It did not come without significant cost. I had this opportunity because:

- God has provided me with 60+ years of healthy life.
- I have trained as a ninja for three-plus years and well over 1,000 hours.
- I have spent hundreds of dollars on obstacles and training equipment for my home.
- I have spent many hours and dollars competing in ninja competitions across the United States.
- I have built hundreds of ninja relationships that helped open the door to the early walk-on line.
- I am retired and have the freedom and time to go to a walk-on line and be in it for 16 days.

- God has blessed us financially, enabling us to have a "Blessing Money" fund that, with my wife's support, helped cover the expenses of being in the walk-on line.
- My coaching clients were willing to slide their scheduled coaching sessions.
- Tim and Bonnie were willing to house me while I was in line.
- I was willing to stick with it and endure the requirements and challenges, including the check-ins, being sick, going through an injury, and so much more.
- I made the decision to leave when I did to solidify my number-10 spot in the line. Only 12 walk-on-line ninjas were given the opportunity to run in Cleveland.
- I remained ready to do whatever I needed to until and during the moment I competed on the course.

I am so thankful for each of these contributions to the opportunity.

My Four Priorities

This experience was an investment. I believe it was a great investment when I consider my core values. It met all four of my priorities for how I want to invest my remaining time on this earth. They are:
- Create memorable experiences.
- Deepen relationships and develop new ones.
- Learn and grow.

- Contribute to others.

This experience created many new memories for me. It gave me the opportunity to meet many new people and take some existing relationships even deeper. It gave me a chance to learn a lot about the *ANW* process. It helped me see how I handle challenges and that I was able to push through when things got hard. And finally it gave me the opportunity to contribute to others by supporting the others in our walk-on line.

Thank you!

Thanks for your engagement and for investing your valuable time in reading *What Just Happened?: The Line*. I hope you enjoyed traveling with me through this crazy experience and that you learned some things that will help you move forward with a challenge or endeavor.

If you enjoyed *What Just Happened?: The Line*, consider passing it on to someone you think would enjoy it or who could benefit from its key messages. It might be a great gift idea for family and friends who just can't get enough of *American Ninja Warrior*. If you would like others to reap the benefits, consider providing a review at Amazon.com.

As always, move and play and make it another great day and week. And keep adding value to life for others, intentionally living a Well Done Life!

Your friend, author, coach, ninja warrior, and fan,
Chris Warnky

Photo Gallery

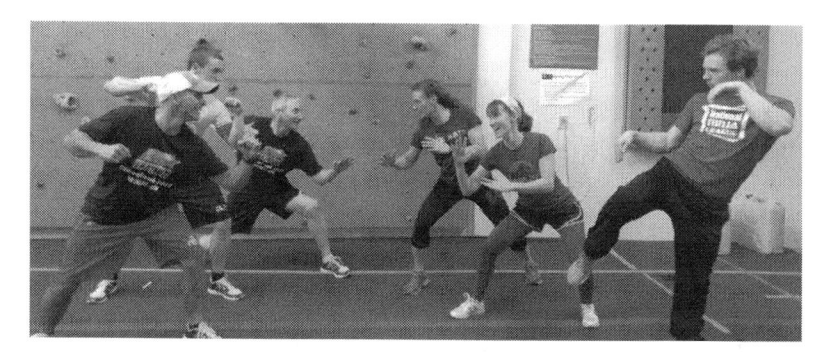

Several from the MLAB OH went to Cleveland to compete on *ANW 9*. On the left are ninjas Scott Walberry, Jesse Wildman, and Chris Warnky, some of our walk-ons; and on the right are Michelle Warnky, Shanon Paglieri, and Sean Noel, some of our invitees.

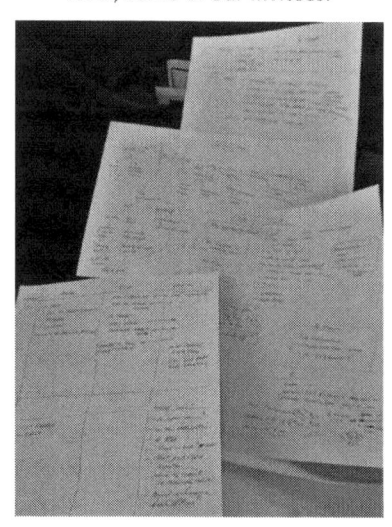

The four sheets of paper I used to evaluate whether or not I should join the walk-on line.

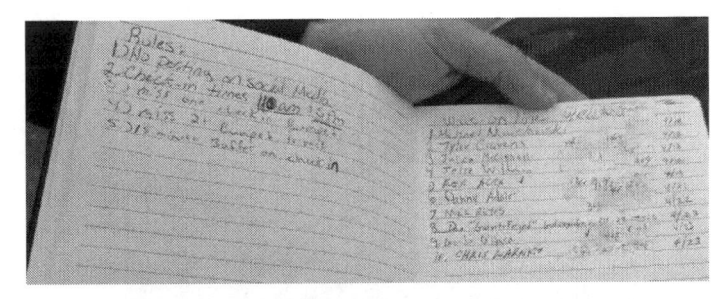

Our walk-on-line sign-in book, just after I signed in.

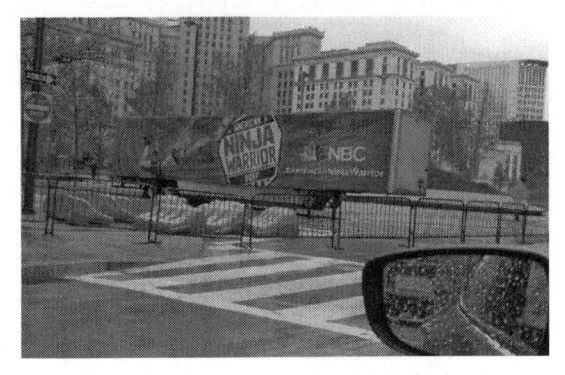

One of the *ANW* trucks that transports the obstacles from city to city. Soon Cleveland would have a full *ANW* obstacle course set up in the center of Public Square.

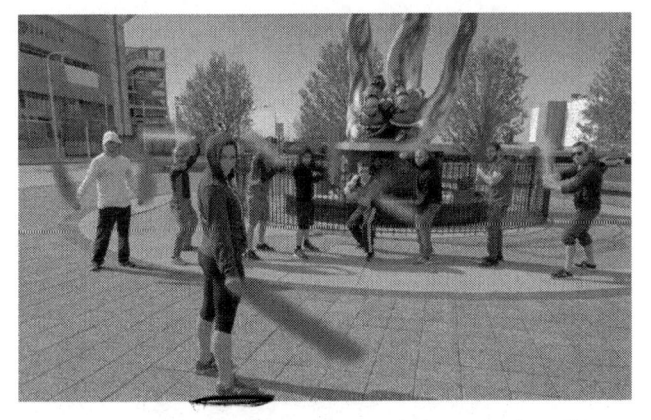

A traditional fun photo as a new ninja joins the line. This was when Brenda joined, just a few hours before I got there.

WHAT JUST HAPPENED?: THE LINE

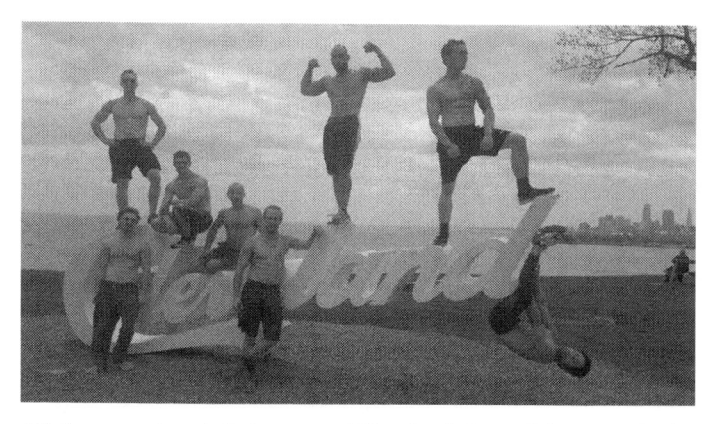

Walk-ons posing at that very cool Cleveland sign at Edgewater Park. Invitee Sean Noel also dropped in for a short visit.

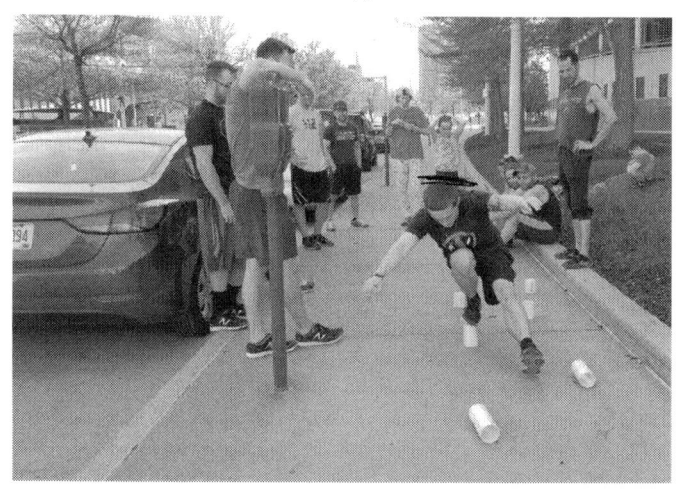

Walk-on-line members playing while waiting to start our next formal check-in. These are some of my obstacles from my car trunk. Go Jesse!

CHRIS WARNKY

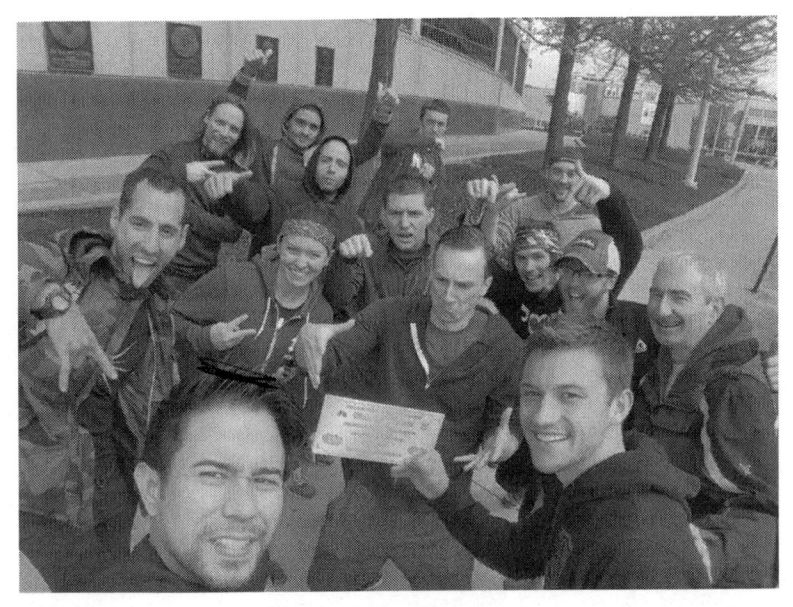

Our walk-on-line check-in after we heard about Michael receiving his Golden Ticket (Michael is holding his valued ticket) to compete on *ANW* in Cleveland, his home town.

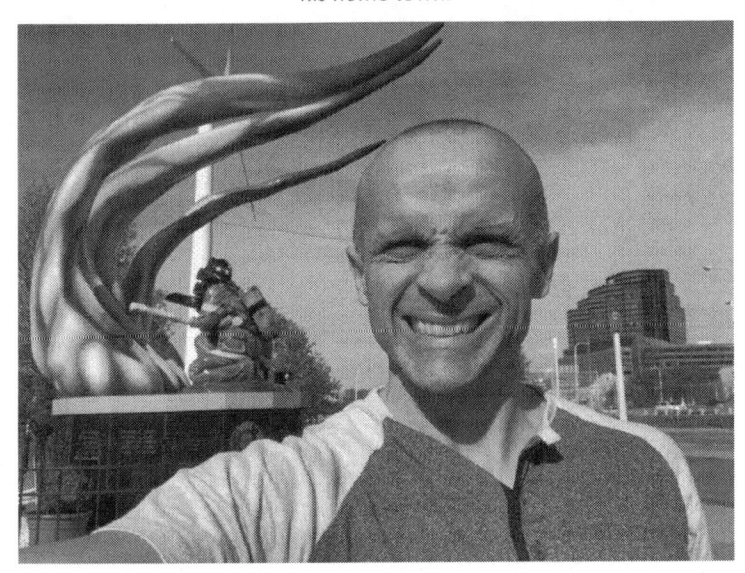

Scott's check-in photo as he joined the line.

WHAT JUST HAPPENED?: THE LINE

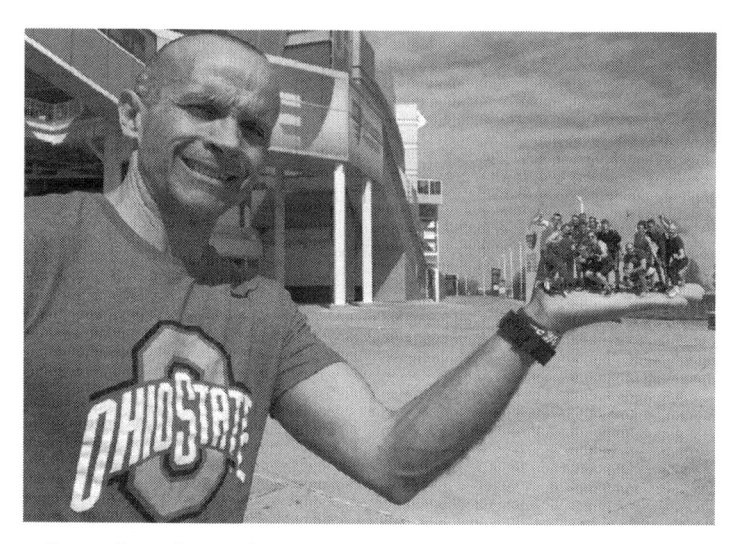

Our walk-on-line traditional group shot when Scott joined our line.

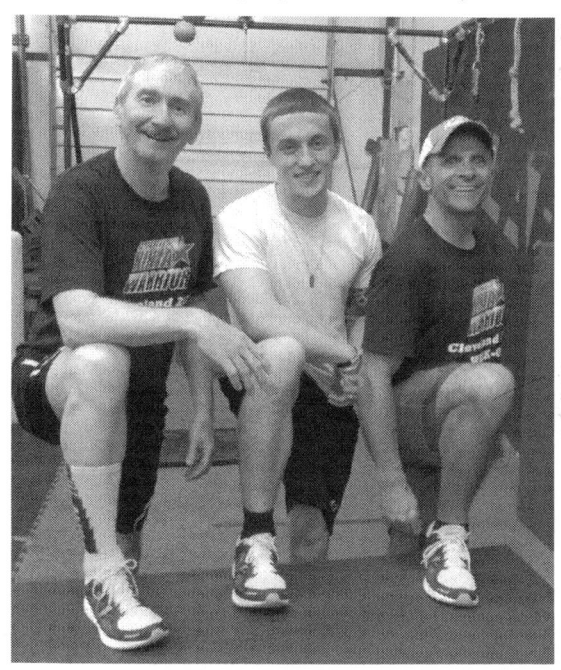

Me with MLAB OH walk-ons Jesse and Scott. We are all wearing the same type and color ninja shoes.

CHRIS WARNKY

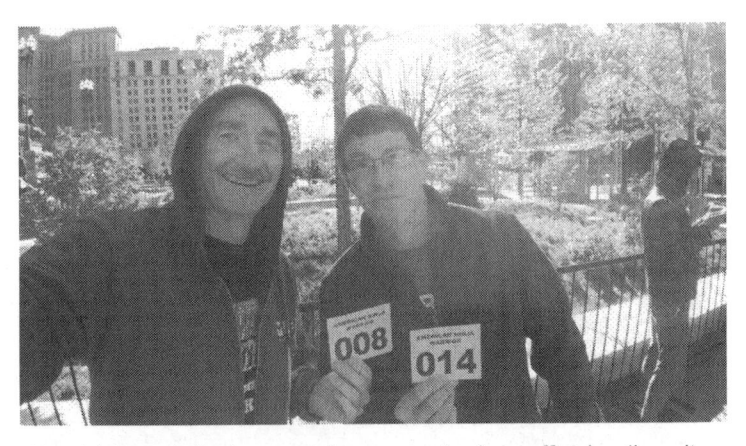

Me with Bryce LaRoche soon after we received our official walk-on-line numbers in the early evening of the city qualifier.

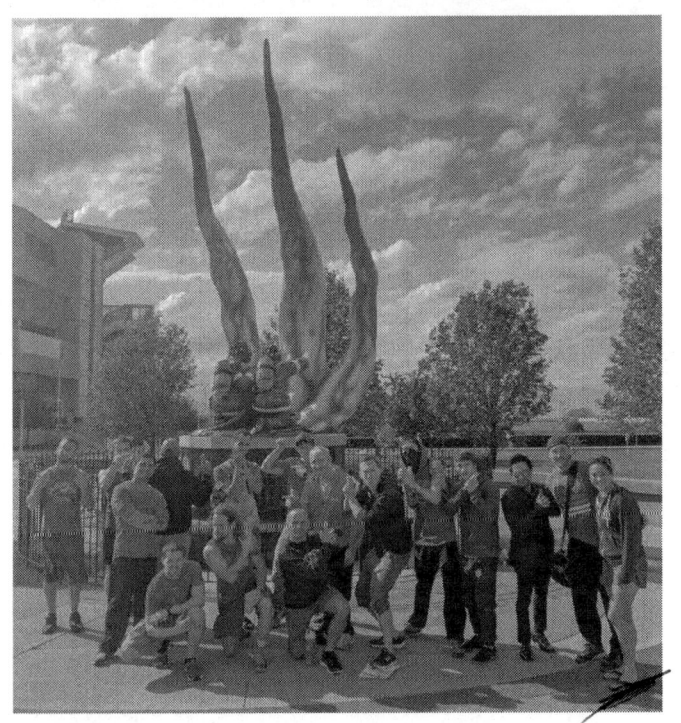

Another walk-on-line group shot – this one in front of the fireman memorial located in front of the Great Lakes Science Center.

WHAT JUST HAPPENED?: THE LINE

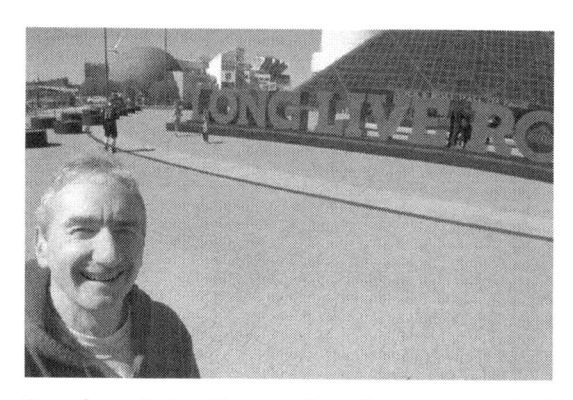

One of our shots with our walk-on line was at the Rock and Roll Hall of Fame on the other side of the Great Lakes Science Center.

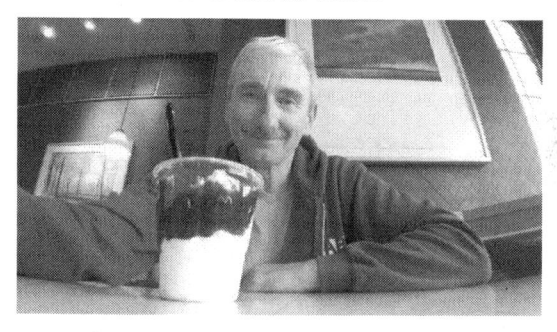

One of those times I had to make another purchase at a fast-food restaurant because I felt guilty about the number of hours I had been there after my meal.

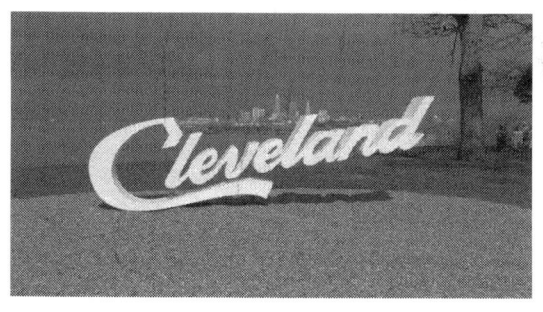

This was when the sun peeked through a small hole in the clouds hitting only the Cleveland sign with amazing light. It looked surreal!

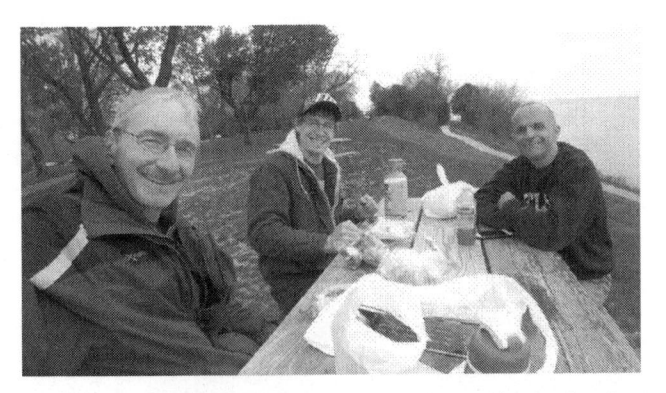

After a supermarket trip, with Bryce and Scott, having lunch next to the lake at Edgewater Park.

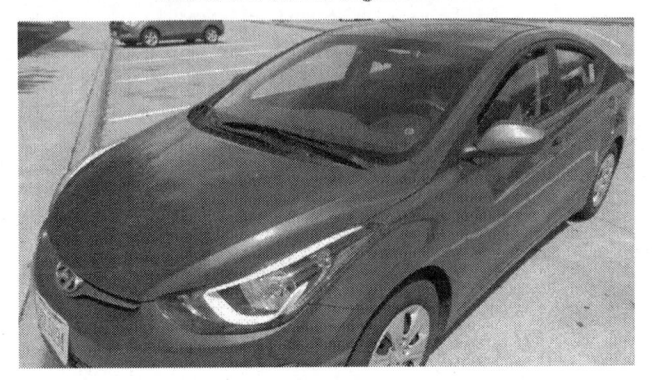

My car was my hotel for much of my time in Cleveland, especially during the day.

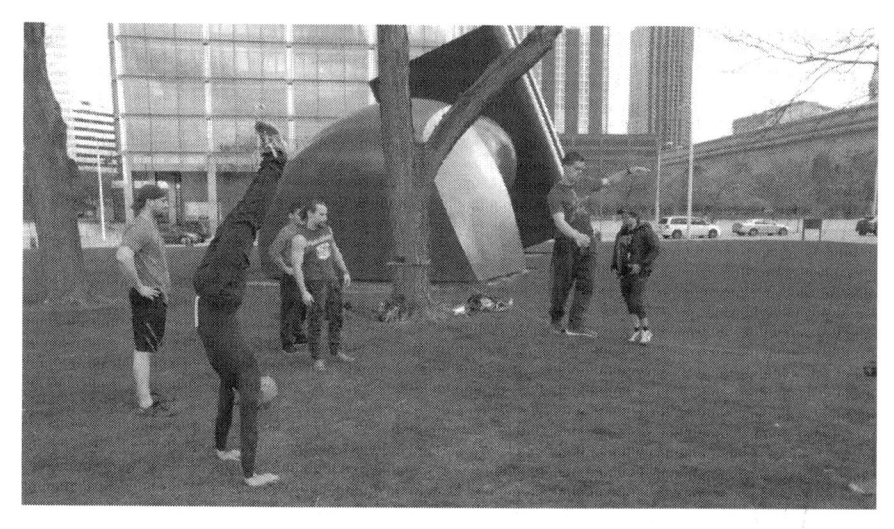

More walk-on-line slacklining at a downtown Cleveland park.

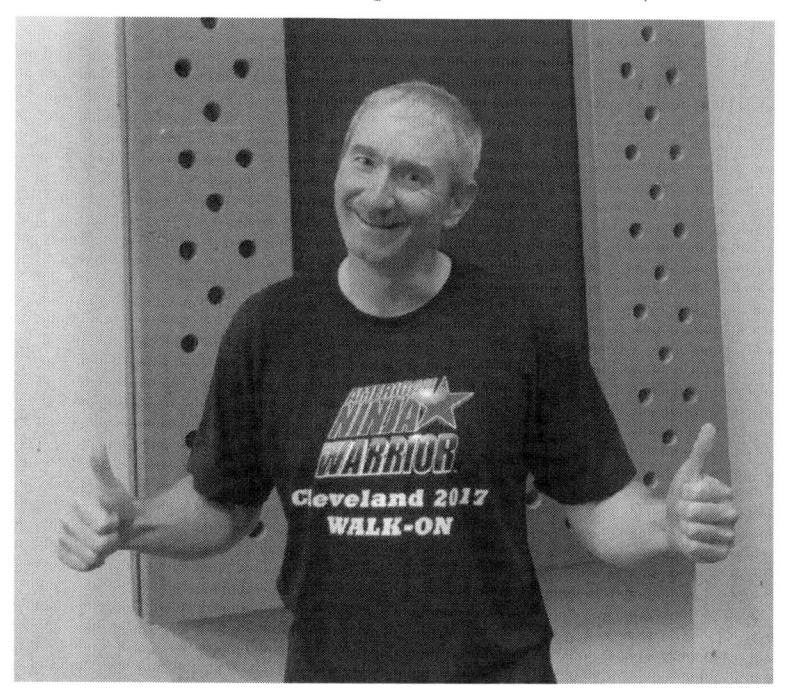

A fun shot we took back at MLAB OH with me wearing my new walk-on-line shirt produced by Scott Reuter.

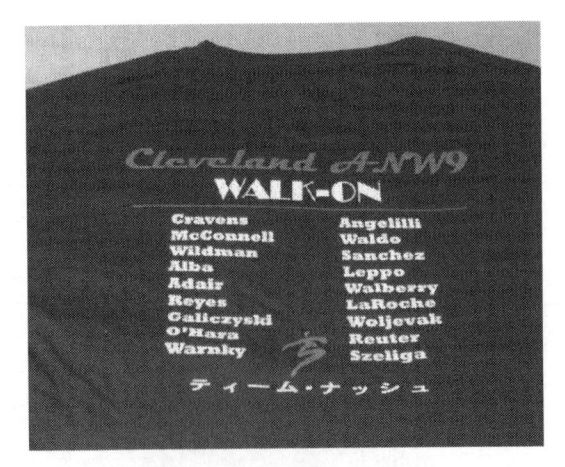

The back of our walk-on-line shirt.

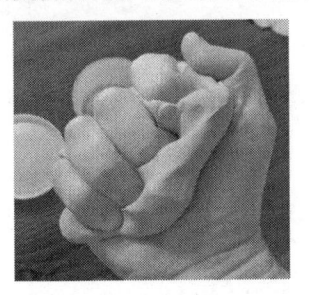

The putty I used to exercise my fingers in the car during drives to and from downtown.

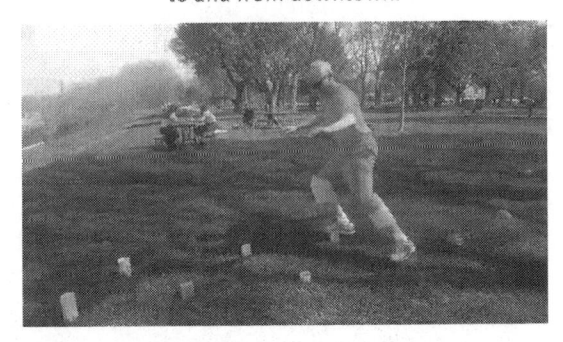

One of the little balance obstacle courses I set up at Edgewater Park. This is close to where I fell on the wooden block on another trip to the park.

WHAT JUST HAPPENED?: THE LINE

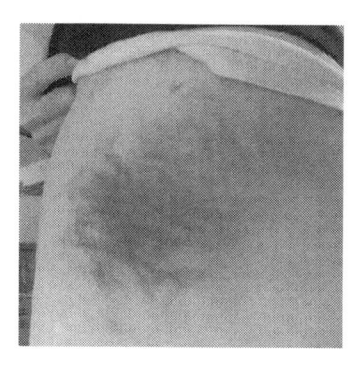

A shot of my hip bruise after it finally started to reveal that stinging on the inside.

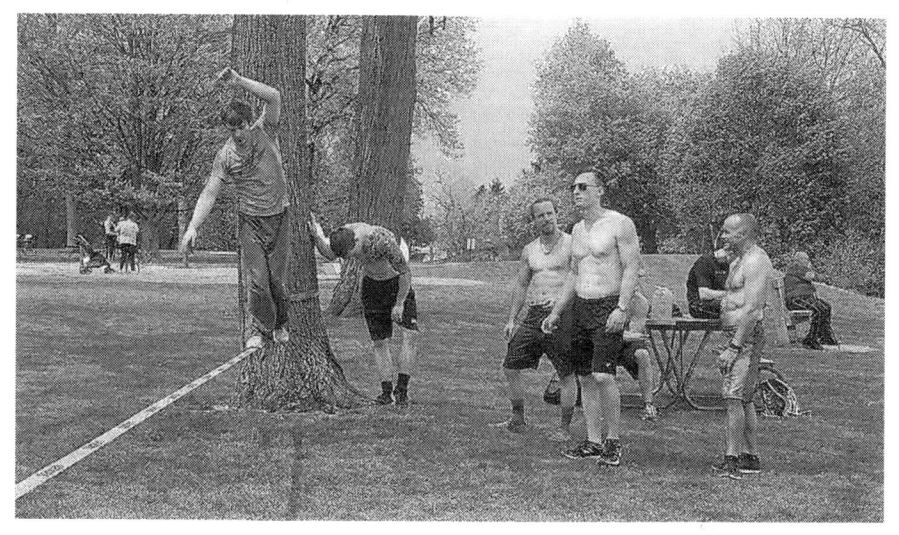

Our walk-on-line ninjas playing on a slack line at Edgewater Park. We were visited by friend and 2017 *ANW* invitee Sean Noel, who is on this slack line.

CHRIS WARNKY

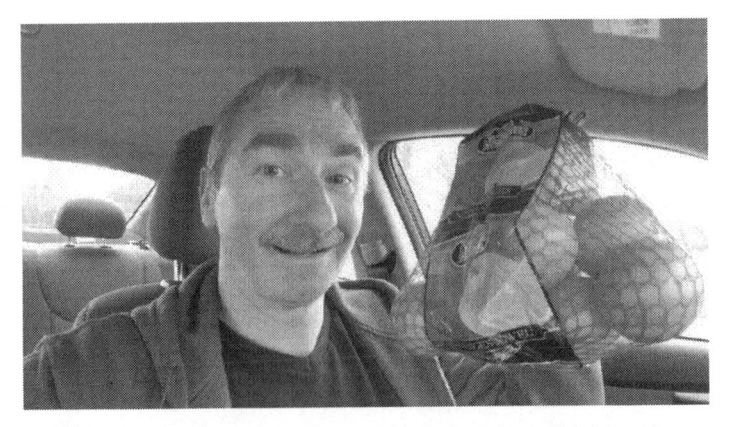

My bag of oranges to see if it would help defeat my bad cold.

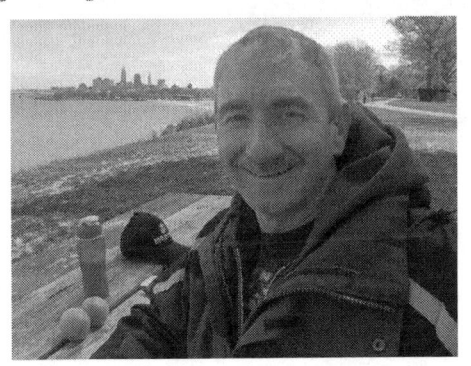

Time to eat another orange or two and not create a mess inside my car.

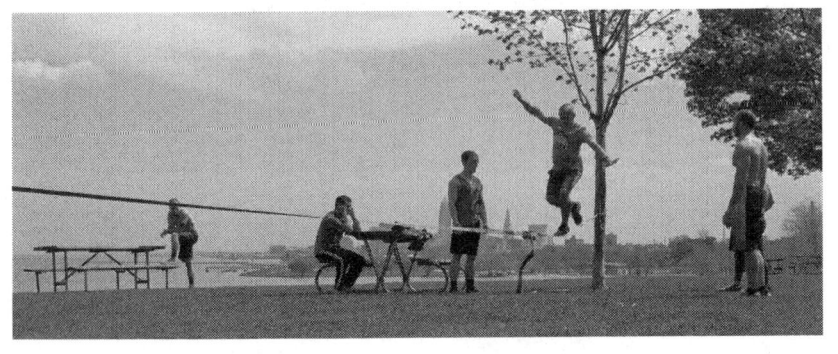

Ninja Scott Walberry testing his slack-line skills at Edgewater Park with the city of Cleveland in the background.

WHAT JUST HAPPENED?: THE LINE

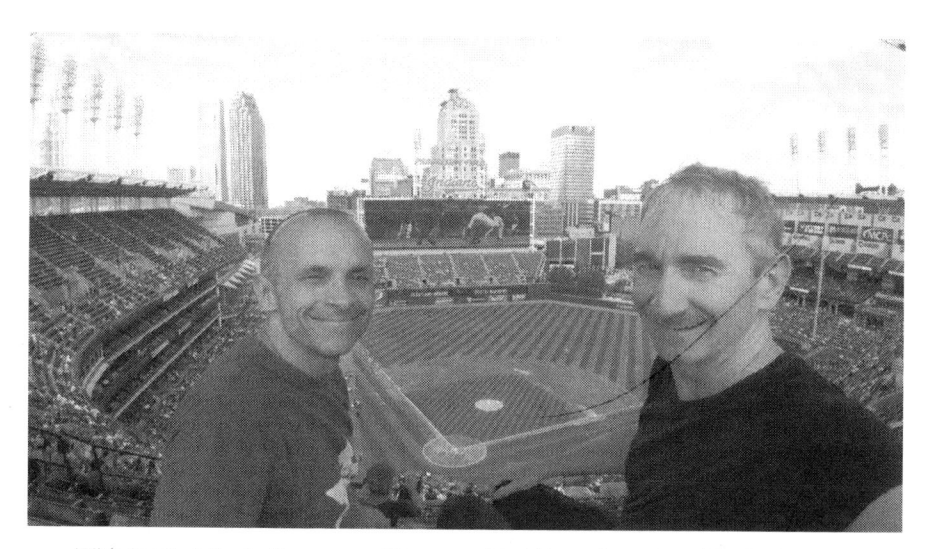

With Scott at the Indians game. They won big. We really enjoyed the break.

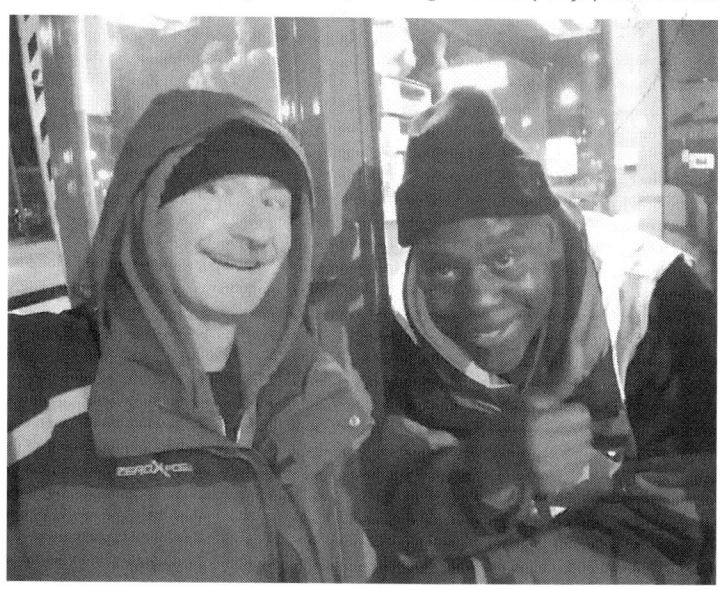

With parking lot attendant Ernie at 5:00 a.m. on the day of our official walk-on-line meet-up with the senior casting producer.

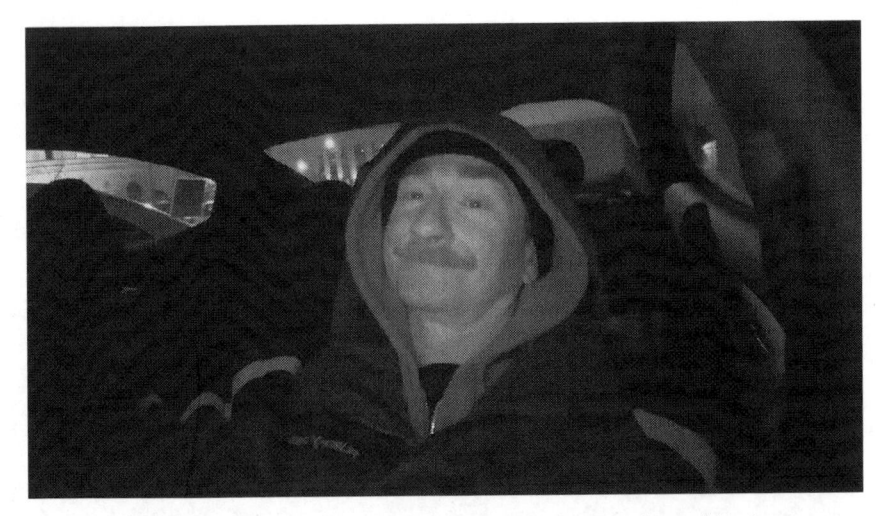

The day the official walk-on line was to form, I am waiting in the parking lot, in my car, for daylight and for the other ninjas to arrive.

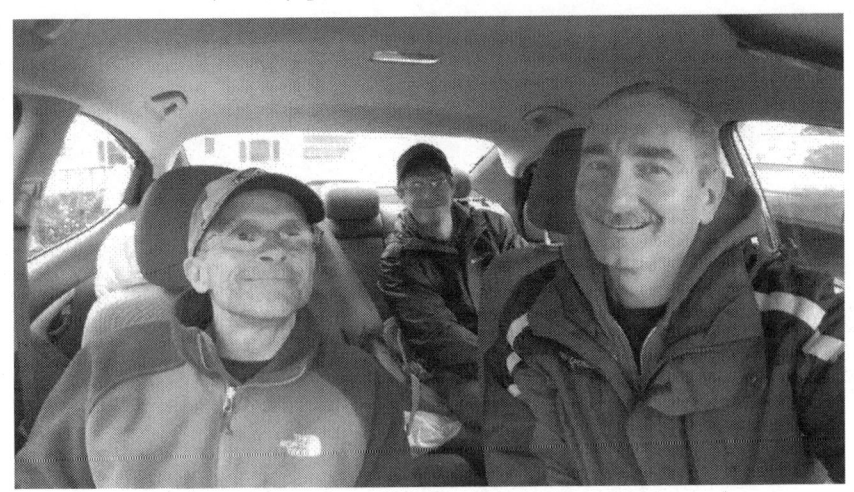

Scott and Bryce join me in my car while we watch additional ninjas enter the parking lot to join the walk-on line that will officially start at 10:00 a.m.

WHAT JUST HAPPENED?: The Line

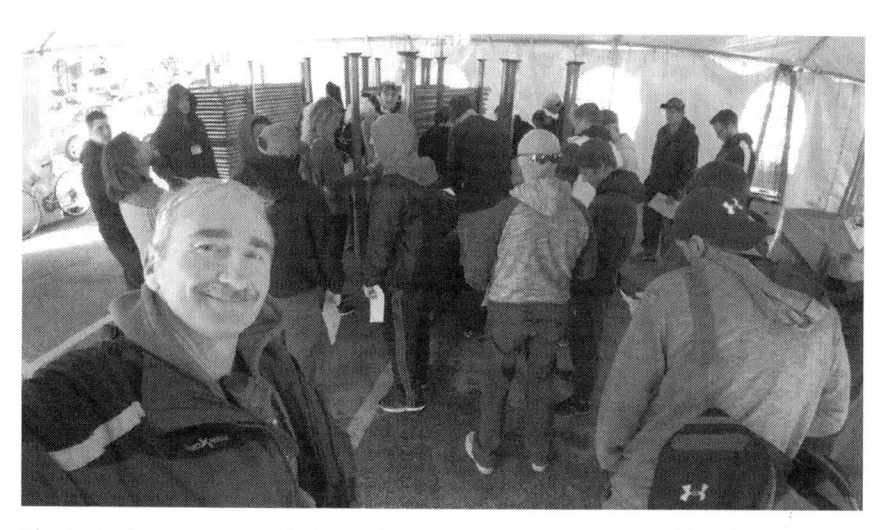

The tent where we met with the senior casting producer, as our walk-on line is made official.

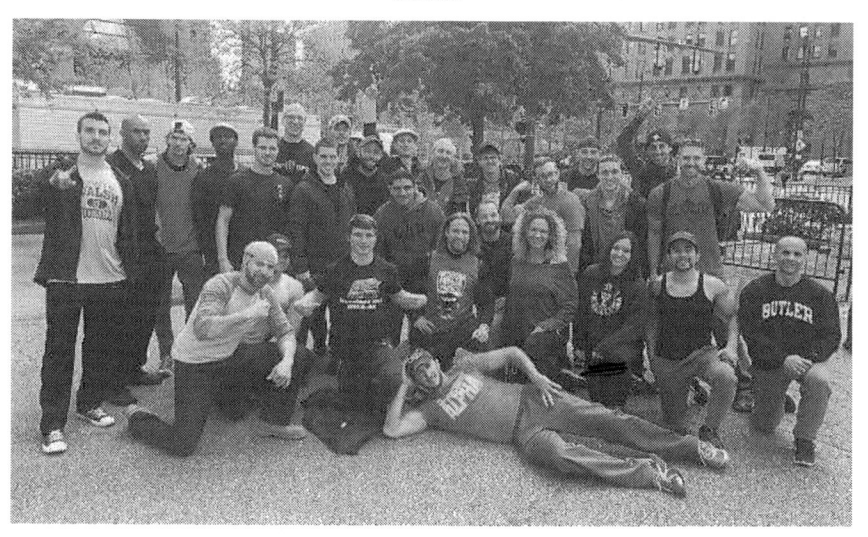

The photo taken by our senior casting producer to document our 2017 *ANW* Cleveland walk-on line. I'm in the middle in the back.

CLEVELAND PUBLIC SQUARE TRAFFIC

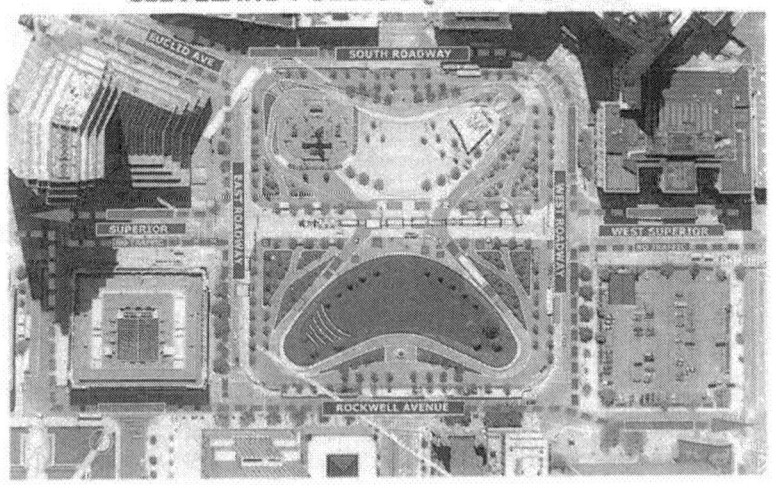

The *ANW* course was set up down the center of Public Square. Our walk-on-line setup for our Sunday shoot was on the terrace just below Superior Ave. E. in this diagram.

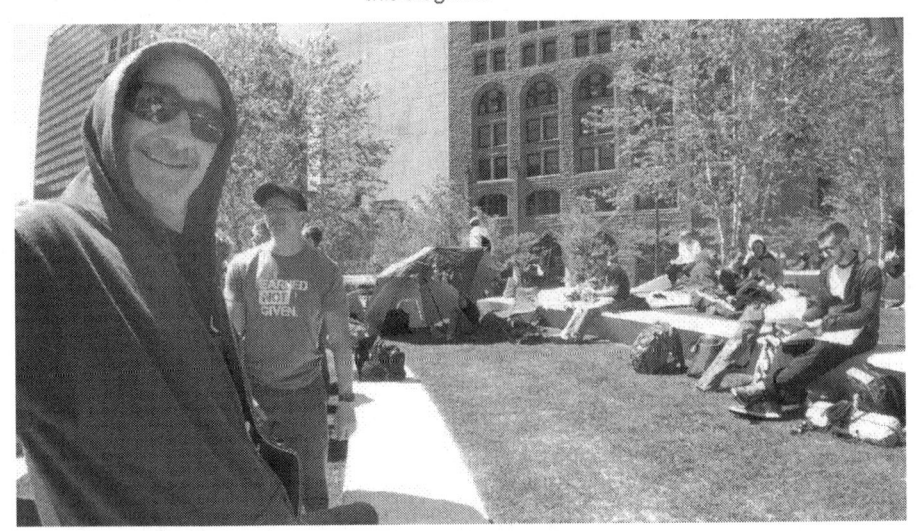

Our Sunday walk-on-line shoot as we were spread across the terrace.

WHAT JUST HAPPENED?: THE LINE

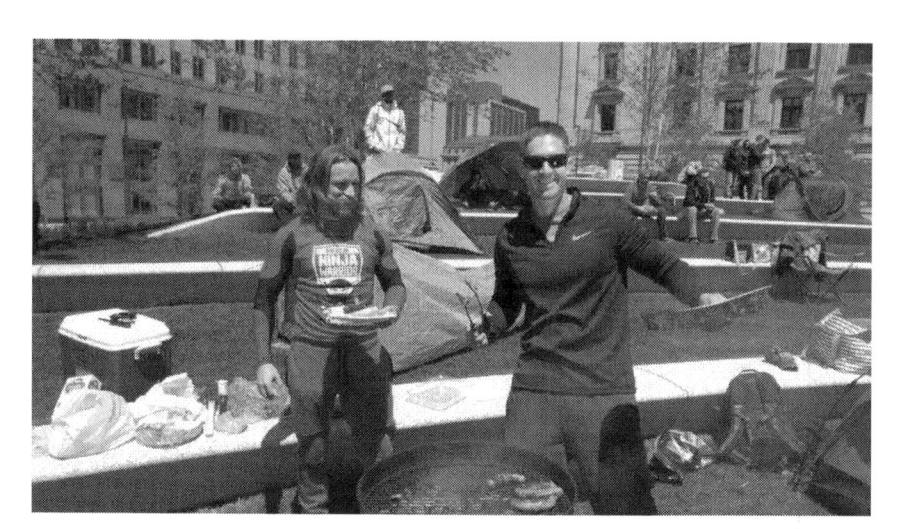

Danny and our cook, ninja Scott Reuter, grilling hot dogs and hamburgers for our walk-on line during our Sunday afternoon video shoot.

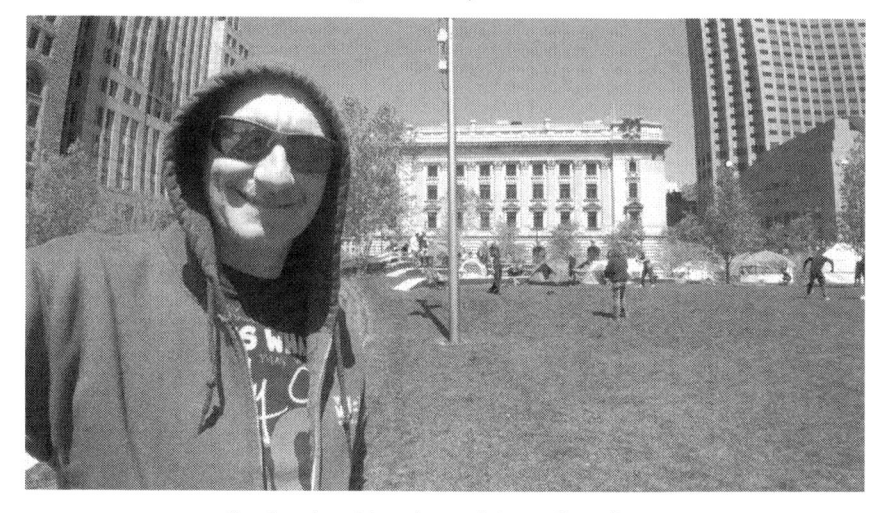

Our Sunday video shoot of the walk-on line.

CHRIS WARNKY

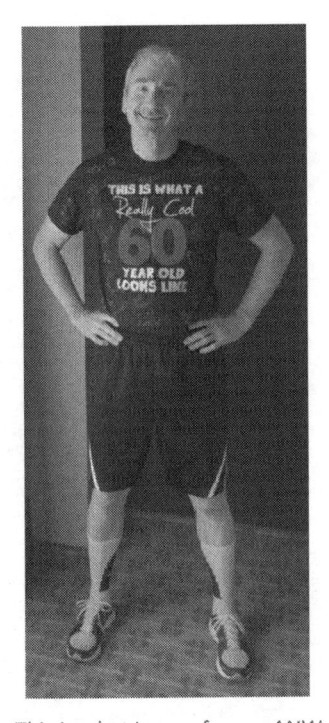

This is what I wore for my *ANW* Cleveland run. I just got dressed and it was time to head to the course.

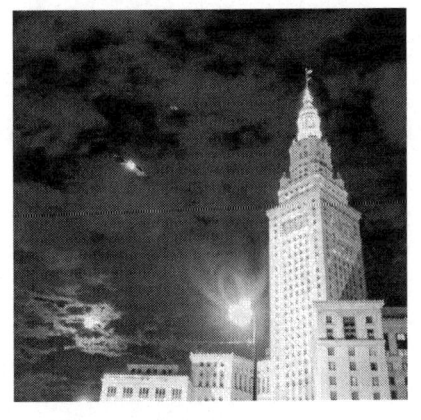

The spectacular Cleveland skyline in the middle of the night of the *ANW* 2017 city qualifier.

WHAT JUST HAPPENED?: THE LINE

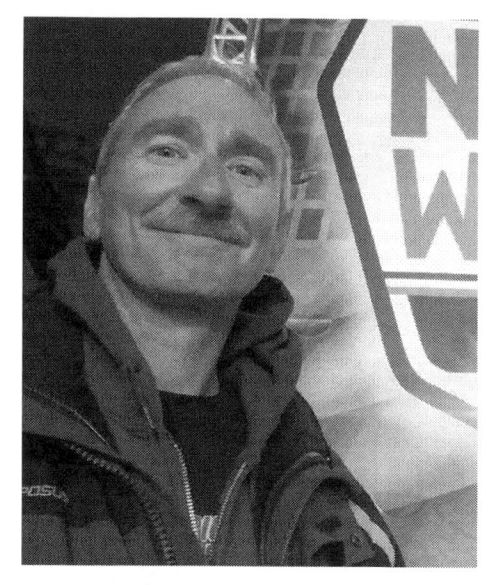

A very thankful guy as this wait was finally over and I was going to be running on the *ANW* course.

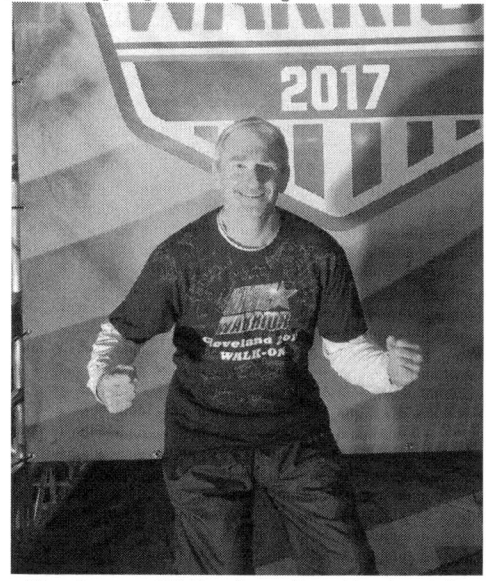

Wearing my *ANW* walk-on-line shirt the night of the city finals.

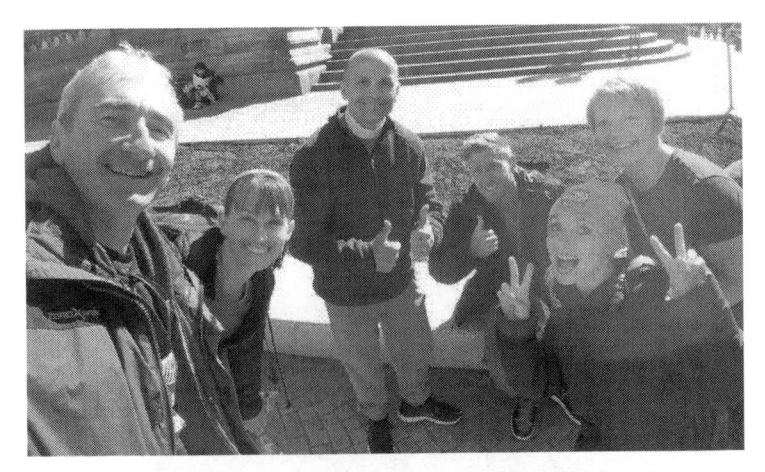

Outside the course on the afternoon of the city qualifier with Shanon, Scott, Cory Cook, Peggy, and Katie.

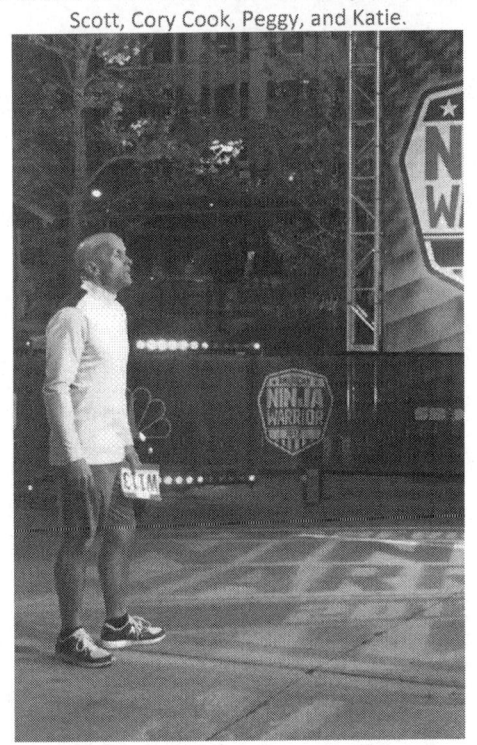

Scott getting ready to go up onto the stage, so close to getting to run, but not this time.

WHAT JUST HAPPENED?: THE LINE

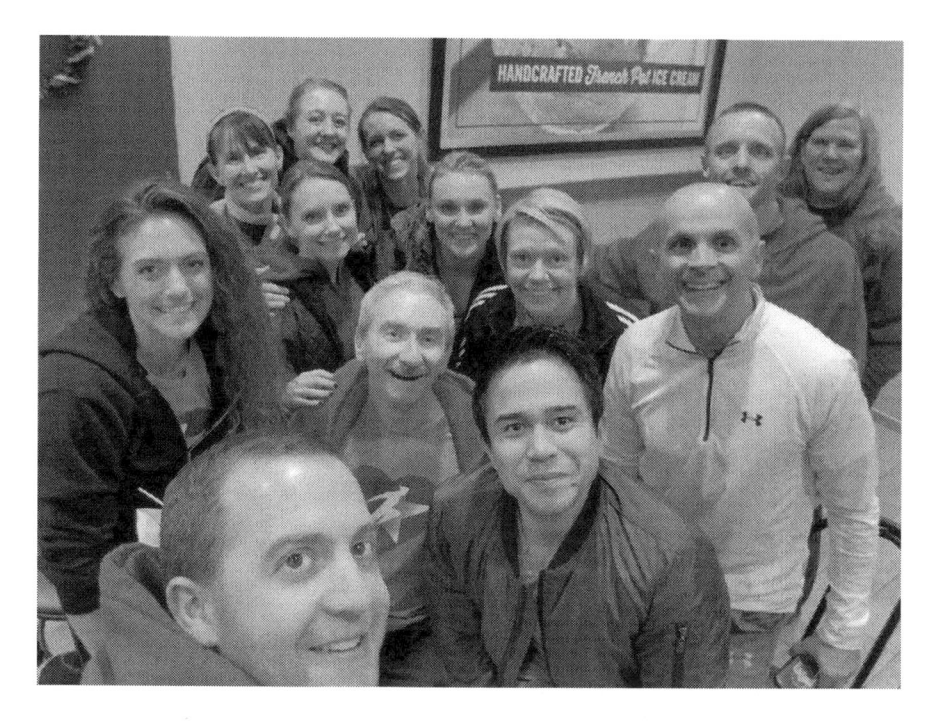

A celebration at Graeter's ice cream shop with a bunch of my MLAB OH ninja buddies as we celebrate the publishing of my first ninja book, The Heart of a Ninja.

Learn More

Contact Information

Chris Warnky, author, ninja competitor, executive and life coach, motivational speaker, and trainer

    Owner, Well Done Life LLC
    Cell phone: 614.787.8591 (call or text)
    Email: chriswarnky@gmail.com
    Facebook: welldonelife
    Web site: welldone-life.com
    Blog: http://cwarnky.wordpress.com

Training as a Ninja

Attend a Ninja Lite session at Movement Lab Ohio with instructor Chris Warnky.

Ask about personal and individualized one-on-one Ninja Lite training sessions with instructor Chris Warnky.

Want Chris to Speak to Your Group?

Chris is available to speak to groups on a variety of topics including:

- Topics in his books
- The Well Done Life Way Coach Approach and materials
- Personal refocus times (retreats)

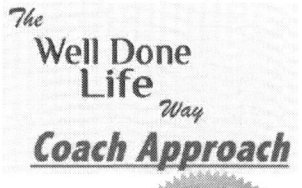

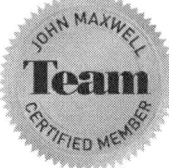

- Leadership and communication topics
- John Maxwell Team Leadership materials

Upcoming Books

These are additional books currently in the works:

- *What Just Happened?: The Run: An American Ninja Warrior Cleveland Course-Run Experience*
- *Refocus Your Life: My Personal Retreat and Assessment Process*
- *The Ten Most Powerful Thoughts and Questions of Your Mind*
- *The Heart of a Ninja for Kids*
- *The Well Done Life® Way Coach Approach to Faster and Better Results*

Get Book Updates

Get added to the email list for book updates by sending "Request for email book updates" to chriswarnky@gmail.com.

Blog updates:

https://cwarnky.wordpress.com/2017/07/06/chris-warnky-books-on-the-way

Facebook updates:

https://www.facebook.com/pg/ChrisWarnkyBooks/posts/?ref=page_internal

Website updates:

https://cwarnky.wixsite.com/chriswarnkybooks

Thirteen percent of initial profits from sales of What Just Happened? *will be donated to Mission Aviation*

Fellowship (MAF), and subsequent profits to MAF and additional charities.

Free Offers

If you would like to receive any of the following free gifts, please request them at chriswarnky@gmail.com:

- Short video greeting from Chris with a bonus ninja training experience story
- Bonus story about Chris's 2017 NNL announcing experience
- Coaching Life Assessment Wheel
- Well Done Life® Way S.M.A.R.T. Goal Development form
- List of Chris's favorite influential books

Be Mentored by Chris Using the 12 Traits of a Ninja

Chris offers "Twelve Trait Mentoring" (from his book *The Heart of a Ninja*), which has been especially ideal for young people who love *American Ninja Warrior* and can benefit from a strong male presence in their lives. Sessions can be conducted in person, by phone, or via Facetime. Choose from 30-, 45-, and 60-minute sessions.

Be Coached by Chris

Chris provides both life coaching and executive coaching.

Learn More about Coaching or Becoming a Coach

Chris offers The Well Done Life Way Coach Approach – over 25 personalized, one-on-one, one-hour courses for those who would like to learn more about how to use coaching to gain faster and better results in their lives.

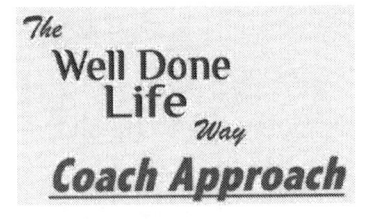

Acknowledgments

First and foremost I'm thankful to our Creator/God for allowing me to live this first 62 years and for providing me with many great relationships and experiences. I am also thankful to have peace with Him because of the life and sacrifice of His Son, Jesus. I am thankful with all of my heart.

Thanks Carolyn, my wife, for your support during the time I invested in learning about, writing, editing, and publishing this and my other books. You are my love. I can't imagine going through anything without you by my side to celebrate our successes and support me in my times of failure and disappointment. I love you!

Thanks to the ninjas who supported me during our two-plus weeks in the Cleveland walk-on line. This includes Julien McConnell, Tyler Cravens, Jesse Wildman, Dan Galiczynski, Brenda O'Hara, Noel Reyes, Danny Adair, Tommy Daly, Jonathan Angelilli, Joshua Sanchez, Scott Walberry, Steve Leppo, and Bryce LaRoche. I appreciate all of you.

There are so many others I am thankful to because of their contributions to my life and/or for their specific help with the writing, editing, and feedback on this book. Below are a few of them:

Thanks to Tim and Bonnie for all the hospitality you provided while I was living in the Cleveland area. Your bed felt so good each night and I highly valued the time I was able to spend with you and your kids, especially in the mornings before I headed to my check-ins.

Thanks, Michelle, for continually supporting me during my ninja journey. I love you so much.

Thanks to my friend and ninja training partner Shanon Paglieri, who has been there most of the way through my entire ninja training. It has been a ball to be able to enjoy this ride together. Thanks for your many encouragements and for your recommendations for this book.

Thanks, Scott Walberry, for your friendship and ongoing support. I always enjoy training with you at MLAB OH. I love to cheer you on anytime you compete. You are amazing. It was great to be able to have you alongside as we walked through much of this ninja walk-on-line experience together. Thanks for allowing me to share the heartfelt letter you shared with your Facebook friends following your disappointment in not getting to run the course. You are an amazing man. Thanks for being one of my beta readers for this book and for your insights, suggestions, and support, and thanks for writing the foreword for this book.

In addition to Shanon and Scott, thanks to my other Lunch Time Training Partners (LTTPs) Chad Kohler and Rex Alba, who support me weekly as we train and compete together. Thanks also to LTTP Katie Tennant, who along with Scott Walberry has been a regular at our noon open gym sessions during the summer and during the school year when your work schedule allows. Thanks also to so many other MLAB OH ninjas I train with. I love spending time with all of you.

I'm very thankful for all the great support and instruction provided by the MLAB OH instructors, especially those who have been there for so many lunchtime open gyms and ninja classes. These include head instructors Jesse Wildman (also a walk-on-line teammate), Kyle Wheeler, Justin Allen, and Sophia Oster. You add so much value to the training for me and others. I appreciate you.

Thanks, ninja-walk-on-line experts Julien McConnell, Greg Schwartz, Yancey Quezada, and David Kavanagh. You have each been in so many *ANW* walk-on lines over the years and your knowledge was very helpful in writing this book.

Thanks to the many ninjas across the country who have welcomed and embraced me into your community. Thank you so much for the encouragement, support, and friendship, and the tips you provided to make me a better ninja. I appreciate you.

Thanks finally to Gwen Hoffnagle, my professional editor for my first two ninja books. You have taken my original manuscript to new and much higher levels. I enjoy working with you and appreciate the value you provide. I would recommend you to any author as long as they don't bump me in line when I want to employ your services. Thank you so much!

About the Author

Chris Warnky is 62 years young and has been married to his love, Carolyn May Warnky, for over 39 years. He has two children: Tim, who lives in Cleveland with his wife, Bonnie, and two daughters; and Michelle, who lives in Columbus and is a popular six-year *American Ninja Warrior* competitor and a serious, competitive obstacle-course racer.

Chris is an active, training ninja warrior dedicated to his Lunch Time Training Partners. He is also an MLAB OH Ninja Lite class instructor and offers personal one-on-one ninja-lite-level targeted training sessions.

He competed in the 2017 *American Ninja Warrior* Cleveland city qualifier and has competed in numerous ninja competitions over the past couple of years including both National Ninja League and Ultimate Ninja Athlete Association competitions. He provided the play-by-play for numerous Facebook Livestream ninja competitions, including the NNL finals.

Chris has been a Bible-reading and believing Christian for over 50 years. His relationship with God is the basis for his life.

He is an author with plans to write several additional books, a professional executive and life coach, and a thought-provoking speaker through his business, Well Done Life. He coaches clients addressing important life and business topics.

Chris is a certified coach, speaker, and trainer with the John Maxwell Team. He is a member of the Maxwell Mentorship Team and served two years on the organization's President's Advisory Council. He served two terms as the International Coach Federation Columbus Charter Chapter president. He achieved the Toastmasters International "Competent Communicator" designation.

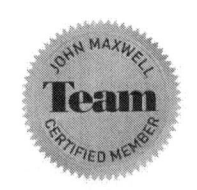

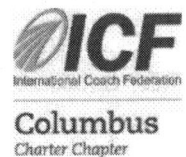

Chris has over three decades of corporate leadership experience, including 23 years as a vice president at Bank One/JP Morgan Chase contributing as a project manager, program manager, and compensation manager.

Made in the USA
Lexington, KY
17 February 2019